Drugs: A Very Short Introduction

'a slim but assured and wise volume on drugs. [It] takes up many controversial positions . . . with an air of authority that commands respect. It is difficult to think of a better overview of the field for anyone new to it.'
David Healy, University of Wales College of Medicine

'a fascinating account of the ways that drugs have been developed, of how they work and of their therapeutic effects . . . admirably succinct and easy to read.'
Lord Walter Perry, The Open University of Scotland

'. . . achieves within a short space an account of the history, the main features of the most commonly used drugs and a peer into the future written in a lively and easily comprehended style.'
Sir Arnold Burgen, Downing College, Cambridge

VERY SHORT INTRODUCTIONS are for anyone wanting a stimulating and accessible way in to a new subject. They are written by experts, and have been published in more than 25 languages worldwide.

The series began in 1995, and now represents a wide variety of topics in history, philosophy, religion, science, and the humanities. Over the next few years it will grow to a library of around 200 volumes – a Very Short Introduction to everything from ancient Egypt and Indian philosophy to conceptual art and cosmology.

Very Short Introductions available now:

ANCIENT PHILOSOPHY
  Julia Annas
THE ANGLO-SAXON AGE
  John Blair
ANIMAL RIGHTS   David DeGrazia
ARCHAEOLOGY   Paul Bahn
ARCHITECTURE
  Andrew Ballantyne
ARISTOTLE   Jonathan Barnes
ART HISTORY   Dana Arnold
ART THEORY   Cynthia Freeland
THE HISTORY OF
  ASTRONOMY   Michael Hoskin
ATHEISM   Julian Baggini
AUGUSTINE   Henry Chadwick
BARTHES   Jonathan Culler
THE BIBLE   John Riches
BRITISH POLITICS
  Anthony Wright
BUDDHA   Michael Carrithers
BUDDHISM   Damien Keown
CAPITALISM   James Fulcher
THE CELTS   Barry Cunliffe
CHOICE THEORY
  Michael Allingham
CHRISTIAN ART   Beth Williamson
CLASSICS   Mary Beard and
  John Henderson
CLAUSEWITZ   Michael Howard
THE COLD WAR
  Robert McMahon

CONTINENTAL PHILOSOPHY
  Simon Critchley
COSMOLOGY   Peter Coles
CRYPTOGRAPHY
  Fred Piper and Sean Murphy
DADA AND SURREALISM
  David Hopkins
DARWIN   Jonathan Howard
DEMOCRACY   Bernard Crick
DESCARTES   Tom Sorell
DRUGS   Leslie Iversen
THE EARTH   Martin Redfern
EGYPTIAN MYTHOLOGY
  Geraldine Pinch
EIGHTEENTH-CENTURY
  BRITAIN   Paul Langford
THE ELEMENTS   Philip Ball
EMOTION   Dylan Evans
EMPIRE   Stephen Howe
ENGELS   Terrell Carver
ETHICS   Simon Blackburn
THE EUROPEAN UNION
  John Pinder
EVOLUTION
  Brian and Deborah Charlesworth
FASCISM   Kevin Passmore
THE FRENCH REVOLUTION
  William Doyle
FREUD   Anthony Storr
GALILEO   Stillman Drake
GANDHI   Bhikhu Parekh

Available soon:

For more information visit our web site

www.oup.co.uk/vsi

Leslie Iversen

DRUGS

A Very Short Introduction

OXFORD
UNIVERSITY PRESS

OXFORD

UNIVERSITY PRESS

Great Clarendon Street, Oxford OX2 6DP

Oxford University Press is a department of the University of Oxford.
It furthers the University's objective of excellence in research, scholarship,
and education by publishing worldwide in

Oxford New York

Auckland Bangkok Buenos Aires Cape Town Chennai
Dar es Salaam Delhi Hong Kong Istanbul Karachi Kolkata
Kuala Lumpur Madrid Melbourne Mexico City Mumbai Nairobi
São Paulo Shanghai Taipei Tokyo Toronto

Oxford is a registered trade mark of Oxford University Press
in the UK and in certain other countries

Published in the United States
by Oxford University Press Inc., New York

British Library Cataloguing in Publication Data
Data available

Library of Congress Cataloging in Publication Data
Data available
ISBN 978-0-19-285431-5

9 10

Typeset by RefineCatch Ltd, Bungay, Suffolk
Printed in Great Britain by
Ashford Colour Press Ltd., Gosport, Hants

Contents

List of illustrations

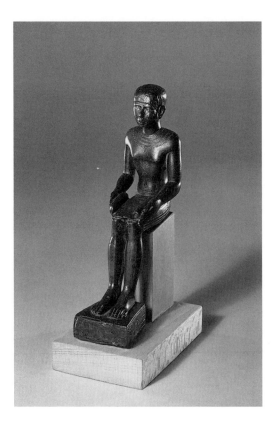

1. Bronze statuette of the god Imhotep. He was an Egyptian doctor, who lived around 2600 BC and was later revered as a god. His treatments included the use of herbs, surgery, and magic. Some of the treatments used have since been shown to have sound medicinal properties; for example, honey has antibacterial properties and was used to heal wounds.

Chapter 1
History

The word 'drug' refers to a chemical substance that is taken deliberately in order to obtain some desirable effect. Some drugs are used medically to treat illnesses whereas others are taken because of their pleasurable effects. Both uses are ancient in their origins. The first humans were hunter-gatherers; they had to learn which of the thousands of plants in their environment were good to eat and which were poisonous. By trial and error they also gradually accumulated knowledge of which plants or other natural materials might help to relieve pain or treat the symptoms of their illnesses. The consumption of medicinal plants is not restricted to humans; studies of chimpanzee behaviour have revealed that sick animals sometimes select plants not usually contained in their diet for their antiparasitic effects.

Before there was a written language, knowledge of plant medicines was handed on by word of mouth from one generation to another. This eventually became a specialized occupation for the 'medicine man', 'shaman', or 'witch doctor', who often combined medical knowledge with the practice of magic and religious rites and became a potent and powerful figure in the community. The belief in spirits that could interfere with life for good or evil, and therefore could cause disease, was almost universal, so it is not surprising that knowledge of drugs was combined with this superstitious role.

Medicine and magic

'Man did not at first regard death and disease as natural phenomena. Common maladies, such as colds or constipation, were accepted as part of existence and dealt with by means of such herbal remedies as were available. Serious and disabling diseases, however, were placed in a very different category. These were of supernatural origin. They might be the result of a spell cast upon the victim by some enemy, visitation by a malevolent demon, or the work of an offended god who had either projected some object – a dart, a stone, a worm – into the body of the victim or had abstracted something, usually the soul of the patient. The treatment then applied was to lure the errant soul back to its proper habitat within the body or to extract the evil intruder, be it dart or demon, by counterspells, incantations, potions, suction, or other means.

Encyclopaedia Britannica (1999)

The first pharmacopoeia

Among the earliest written records of herbal medicines are those from ancient China. The earliest book was the *Shen-Nung Pen T'sao Ching*, published during the Han dynasty in the second century AD; it listed 365 herbal medicines and became an important basis for the development of Chinese medicine. The book was added to many times. A particularly important revision, *Pen T'sao Keng Mu* (the 'Great Pharmacopoeia'), prepared by Li Shin Chen during the Ming dynasty in the sixteenth century, was in fifty-two volumes and listed 1,898 medicines of plant, animal, and mineral origins. Li was one of the first to study drugs scientifically; he personally studied the actions of many traditional remedies. As a result he discarded a lot of useless information and eliminated some toxic preparations. Pharmacology is the scientific study of drugs, so Li could perhaps be called the first pharmacologist.

Herbal medicines continue to be important in modern Chinese medicine, and many active substances have been introduced into Western medicine from these sources. In Chinese medicine various drugs are mixed and prepared in complex prescriptions according to philosophical principles, to restore the harmony of the yin and the yang and the balance between the five organs, the five planets, and the five colours. The art of prescribing Chinese remedies is complex, and is very different from the use of drugs in modern Western medicine, in which single pure chemical substances are used to treat particular aspects of illness.

In India, the ancient ayurvedic system of medicine originated as long as 3,000 years ago. It remains widely practised in Asia and it too relies heavily on natural drugs, often in complex mixtures. Unlike the relatively benign and non-toxic effects of most Chinese medicines, however, the ayurvedic approach seems often to be more aggressive – with drug-induced vomiting, purging of the gut with laxatives and enemas, and bleeding as common remedies. A number of medical texts also exist from ancient Egypt (2000–1500 BC), describing the use of many herbal and natural medicines: senna, honey, thyme, juniper, frankincense, cumin and colocynth (for digestion); pomegranate root and henbane (for worms), and also flax, oakgall, pine-tar, manna, bayberry, acanthus, aloe, caraway, cedar, coriander, cypress, elderberry, fennel, garlic, wild lettuce, nasturtium, onion, papyrus, poppy plant, saffron, sycamore, and watermelon.

Systemized herbal pharmacopoeias also emerged independently in other cultures. In Greece Dioscorides published his influential *De materie medica* in AD 55, and this was considered an absolute authority for the next 1,600 years. The father of modern medicine, Hippocrates, founded one of the first schools of 'rational' or 'scientific' medicine, and used several hundred natural medicines. In ancient Rome, Pliny (AD 60) published his *Natural History*, the largest ever compilation of knowledge of herbal and other natural remedies. Herbal medicine flourished elsewhere too, notably in the medieval era in the Arab world and in Europe. The British herbal text written by Nicholas Culpepper (1616–54) was one of the most famous; he combined herbal remedies with astrology.

Culpepper's *Pharmacopoeia*: Comfrey

'This is an herb of Saturn, and I suppose under the sign Capricorn, cold, dry and earthly in quality. The Great Comfrey helpeth those that spit blood, or make a bloody urine. The root boiled in water or wine, and the decoction drank, helps all inward hurts, bruises, wounds, and ulcers of the lungs, and causeth the phlegm that oppresseth them to be easily spit forth. It helpeth the defluxion of rheum from the head upon the lungs, the fluxes of blood or of humours by the belly, womens immoderate courses, as well the reds as the whites, and the running of the reins by what cause soever. A syrup made thereof is very effectual for all those inward griefs and hurts, and the distilled water for the same purpose also, and for out-ward wounds and sores in the fleshy or sinewy part of the body whotsoever, as also to take away the fits of agues, and to allay the sharpness of humours. A decoction of the leaves hereof is available to all the purposes, though not so effectual as the roots. The roots being outwardly applied help fresh wounds or cuts immediately, being bruised and laid thereto; and is special good for ruptures and broken bones; yea, it is said to be so powerful to consolidate and knit together, that if they be boiled with dissevered pieces of flesh in a pot, it will join them together again. It is good to be applied to womens breasts that grow sore by the abundance of milk coming into them; also, to repress the overmuch bleeding of the haemorrhoids, to cool the inflammation of the parts thereabouts, and to give ease of pains. The roots of Comfrey taken fresh, beaten small and spread upon leather, and laid upon any place troubled with the gout, does presently give ease of the pains; and applied in the same manner, giveth ease to pained joints, and profiteth very much for running and moist ulcers, gangrenes, mortifications, and the like, for which it hath often experience been found helpful.'

Nicholas Culpepper (1770 edition)

The era of herbal medicine lasted for many centuries. Herbal remedies included several very potent and effective medicines, but there was also much mythology. According to the 'Doctrine of Signatures', remedies for disease could be recognized by some property or 'signature' that they possessed. For example, cyclamen plants were used to treat disorders of the ear because their leaves were shaped like human ears; saffron because of its yellow colour was used to treat jaundice; and the mandrake plant and ginseng were used for many ailments because their roots often resembled the human form.

The era of scientific medicine

The Renaissance saw the development of a new experimental approach to medicine in the great medical schools of Europe, and the rediscovery of medical knowledge from ancient Greece and Rome. One of the great accomplishments of this era was William Harvey's discovery of the circulation of the blood described in his book *De mortu cordis* (1628).

THE

English Phyſitian

26

ENLARGED:

With Three Hundred, Sixty, and Nine
Medicines made of *Engliſh Herbs* that
were not in any *Impreſsion* until this:
The *Epiſtle* will Inform you how to
know *This Impreſsion* from any other.

Being an *Aſtrologo-Phyſical Diſcourſe* of the *Vulgar
Herbs of this Nation* : *Containing a Compleat Method of Phyſick, whereby a man may preſerve his Body in Health ; or Cure himſelf, being Sick, for three
pence Charge, with ſuch things only as grow in England, they being moſt fit for Engliſh Bodies.*

Herein is alſo ſhewed theſe Seven Things, *viz* 1 The Way of making Plaiſters, Oyntments, Oyls, Pultiſs, Syrups, Decoctions,
Julips, or Waters, of al ſorts of Phyſical Herbs, That you may have
them ready for your uſe at al times of the yeer. 2 What Planet Go-
verneth every Herb or Tree (uſed in Phyſick) that groweth in
England. 3 The Time of gathering al Herbs, both Vulgarly, and
Aſtrologically. 4 The Way of Drying and Keeping the Herbs al
the yeer. 5 The Way of Keeping their Juyces ready for uſe al al
times. 6 The Way of Making and Keeping al kind of uſeful Compounds made of Herbs. 7 The way of mixing *Medicines* according to *Cauſe* and *Mixture* of the *Diſeaſe,* and *Part* of the Body
Afflicted.

By Nich. Culpeper, Gent. Student in *Phyſick*
and *Aſtrologie* : Living in *Spittle Fields.*

London : Printed by Peter *Cole* in *Leaden-Hall,* and are to be ſold
at his Shop at the ſign of the *Printing-preſs in Cornhill,*
neer the *Royal Exchange.* 1653

2. Title page of the 1653 edition of Nicholas Culpepper's pharmacopoeia.
First published in 1616 this became the most famous British herbal text.

Most medical practice, however, continued to rely on traditional remedies, with little regard for scientific evidence. The search for a simple way of healing the sick continued. In eighteenth-century Edinburgh, for example, the writer and lecturer John Brown expounded his view that there were only two diseases, sthenic (strong) and asthenic (weak), and two treatments, stimulant and sedative; his chief remedies were alcohol and opium.

It was not until the nineteenth century that scientific medicine really began to have a major impact on the practice of medicine, led by men like Claude Bernard (1813–78), the famous French physiologist. A key discovery was that infectious diseases were caused by microscopic living organisms. The main credit for this is due to the French chemist Louis Pasteur. It was Pasteur who, by a brilliant series of experiments, proved that the fermentation of wine and the souring of milk are caused by living micro-organisms. His work led to the pasteurization of milk and solved problems of agriculture and industry as well as those of animal and human diseases. He successfully employed inoculations to prevent anthrax in sheep and cattle, chicken cholera in fowl, and finally rabies in humans and dogs.

From Pasteur, Joseph Lister derived the concepts that enabled him to introduce the antiseptic principle into surgery. Up until the mid-century surgical operations and childbirth were associated with a high risk of infection and often death. In 1865 Lister, a professor of surgery at Glasgow University, began placing an antiseptic barrier of carbolic acid between the wound and the germ-containing atmosphere. Infections and deaths fell dramatically, and his pioneering work led to more refined techniques of sterilizing the surgical environment.

William Morton, an American dentist, made surgical operations and childbirth less terrifying by the introduction of ether as an anaesthetic. Another major advance in surgery came from Edinburgh, where the Professor of Midwifery, James Young Simpson, had been experimenting upon himself and his assistants, inhaling various vapours with the object of discovering an effective anaesthetic. In November 1847 chloroform was tried with complete success, and it soon became the anaesthetic of choice. In Britain, official royal sanction was given to anaesthetics by Queen Victoria, who accepted chloroform from her physician, John Snow, when giving birth to her eighth child, Prince Leopold, in 1853.

It was in nineteenth-century Germany, however, that the development of the modern era of drug development began. Germany was a leader in the scientific approach to medicine, and students flocked to German medical schools from all over the world. German chemists were the first to isolate pure drug chemicals from herbal medicines, with the isolation of morphine from crude opium in 1803 and quinine from the bark of the cinchona tree in 1820. Morphine was used as a powerful pain reliever, but, like opium before it, morphine also became a drug of abuse. Quinine had a major impact on the prevention and treatment of malaria. One of the outstanding scientific leaders of that era was Paul Ehrlich. While still a student, Ehrlich carried out work on lead poisoning from which he evolved the theory that was to guide much of his subsequent work – that certain tissues have a selective affinity for certain chemicals. This led in turn to the modern concept that drugs are recognized by specific receptors in the body (see Chapter 2), and indeed Ehrlich was one of the first to use the term 'receptor'. In the early twentieth century J. N. Langley, Professor of Physiology in Cambridge, England, studied the actions of nicotine and the South American arrow poison curare on nerve-muscle preparations, and also concluded that the drugs act on a 'receptive substance' that was neither nerve nor muscle.

Ehrlich experimented with the effects of various chemical substances on disease organisms. In 1910, with his colleague Sahachiro Hata, he conducted successful tests on the 606th compound in a series of synthetic chemicals prepared in his laboratory. The 606th compound

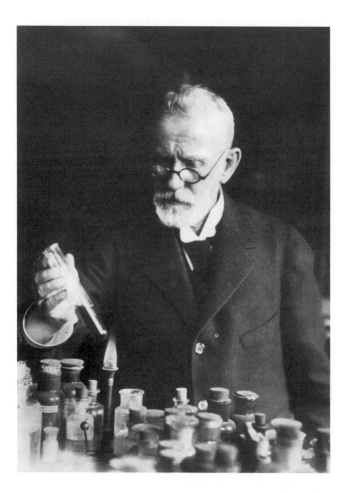

3. Paul Ehrlich, discoverer of Salvarsan and father of modern pharmacology.

was one that contained arsenic and was called arsphenamine. It was one of the first drugs that effectively killed disease micro-organisms, and it inaugurated the era of 'chemotherapy', which was to revolutionize the treatment and control of infectious diseases, which had hitherto been largely untreatable. Arsphenamine (sold under the trade name 'Salvarsan') was particularly lethal to the micro-organism responsible for syphilis. Until the introduction of penicillin, Salvarsan (or one of its close chemical relatives that were subsequently developed) remained the standard treatment of syphilis and went a long way towards bringing this social and medical scourge under control.

German chemists learned how to make synthetic dye chemicals that bound strongly to fabrics and could not be removed by washing. They used the same principles to make synthetic medicines that targeted diseases like 'magic bullets', in Ehrlich's famous phrase. In 1896 Felix Hoffman working for the Bayer company was the first to synthesize aspirin. In 1932 the German bacteriologist Gerhard Domagk discovered that the red dye Prontosil is active against streptococcal infections in mice and humans. Soon afterward French workers showed that its active antibacterial agent is sulphanilamide. In 1936 the English physician Leonard Colebrook and his colleagues provided overwhelming evidence of the efficacy of both Prontosil and sulphanilamide in streptococcal septicaemia (bloodstream infection), thereby ushering in the sulphonamide era. Domagk and others produced new sulphonamides with astonishing rapidity, many of which had greater potency, wider antibacterial range, or lower toxicity. Domagk was awarded the Nobel Prize for Medicine for this work in 1939, but because of his persecution by Nazi Germany he was not able to accept the award until 1947. Some of the new sulpha drugs stood the test of time; others, like the original sulphanilamide and its immediate successor, sulphapyridine, were replaced by safer and more effective successors, many of which are still in use. The sulphonamides represented the first big advance in the war against infectious diseases, which culminated in the development of the antibiotics (see Chapter 6).

The last half of the twentieth century saw an unprecedented flourishing of basic medical research and a remarkable increase in the kinds and numbers of drugs available for clinical use. The list of disease conditions that could be treated expanded enormously, and the discovery and production of new drugs for sale became a major industry. Annual sales of medical drugs in the USA, for example, increased from $149 million in 1939 to $130 billion in 1999 – an increase of nearly a thousandfold. The impact that these new medicines have had on human life and well-being has been extraordinary (see Chapter 6).

Our love affair with recreational drugs

As a species we have a unique propensity to seek out mind-altering chemicals and sometimes to persist in their use even when we know that such behaviour may be damaging to our health. Animals also seem to enjoy intoxicants. For example, apes in the wild will get mildly drunk on over-ripe fruit that has fermented to produce alcohol. My cats enjoy their Christmas treat of a small cloth mouse stuffed with the dried leaves of catmint (Nepeta); they roll wildly on the floor chewing fiercely on this toy and inhaling the intoxicating vapours. But apes do not allow the search for over-ripe fruit to dominate their lives, and my cats do not seek out a regular supply of catmint, even though it is available in our garden.

The recreational use of drugs seems to have been a part of human behaviour for many thousands of years. Alcohol was probably the first such drug – it is easily available from fruit and wild yeasts that are common in most parts of the world. It was a small step to discover how to control the process of fermentation to make wines and beer. There are records of organized drinking houses in ancient Babylon more than 3,000 years ago, and wine making was common in all parts of the Roman Empire. The production of alcoholic drinks in their almost infinite variety has become a large industry, and their consumption, except in Islamic countries, is widespread around the world. Like many other recreational drugs, alcohol has also been widely used in medicine – as a rough and ready anaesthetic in the era before ether and chloroform and as an ingredient in many patent medicines – including gripe water (a dilute sugary alcoholic drink) for restless babies with colic. Alcohol also plays a role in various religions, as in the communion wine of Christianity. The excessive use of alcohol and the liability to dependence came into special prominence in the deprived cities of the industrial era of the nineteenth and twentieth centuries, and most countries reacted by placing restrictive laws on the sale of alcohol and by taxing it heavily.

Smoking tobacco in its various forms is the second most popular form of recreational drug use in the Western world today. The tobacco plant *Nicotiana rustica* is native to North America, and smoking the dried leaves was a custom among many of the American Indian tribes. Smoking formed an important part of Indian ceremonies, such as the smoking of the pipe of peace, and they also believed that tobacco possessed medicinal properties. Christopher Columbus brought the plant and the habit to Europe and it spread rapidly. The early European colonists in America grew tobacco for export to Europe, and it rapidly became the chief commodity of their trade. The cigarette, as a convenient, efficient, and disposable smoking device, was not common until the twentieth century. Cigarette smoking then rose dramatically in popularity, until more than half American men were regular smokers by mid-century, consuming an average of 15–20 cigarettes each day. Ironically, the tobacco companies at first advertised the health benefits of cigarette smoking. It was not until the 1950s that the health risks of tobacco smoking first became apparent, following the pioneering work of Richard Doll and Richard Peto in Oxford. Although the active ingredient in tobacco, nicotine, is relatively non-toxic, the smoke inhaled from burning tobacco leaves is damaging because it contains various chemicals that can trigger cancer – particularly lung cancer.

In India and in the Arab world, smoking the burning leaves of another

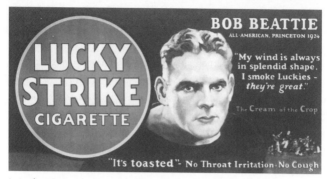

4. In the 1920s advertisements for cigarettes conveyed a healthy message.

plant, *Cannabis sativa*, has been widely practised for thousands of years. The dried leaves ('marijuana') and the more potent female flowering heads of the plant ('sinsemilla') or the sticky cannabis resin can be smoked or consumed in a variety of foodstuffs. In the Hindu religion cannabis plays an important ritual role, and in Islamic countries, where the use of alcohol is forbidden, cannabis use – which is not explicitly mentioned in the Koran – has tended to take its place. The use of cannabis as a recreational drug was virtually unknown in the West until the mid-twentieth century, when it became popular with the beat and hippie generation of the 1960s and 1970s. Since then it has become firmly embedded in Western youth culture, as the third most widely consumed recreational drug after alcohol and tobacco. Plant-breeders in California and in Holland have developed new strains of cannabis plant with an enhanced content of the active ingredient, Δ^9-tetrahydrocannabinol (THC), and there are moves in several Western countries to make cannabis more freely available. Apart from its intoxicant effects, cannabis also has a number of potentially important medicinal uses, and has been widely used in Indian medicine for many centuries. It was also used in Western medicine for almost 100 years from the mid-nineteenth century until the mid-twentieth century, and

13

in the new millennium there are increasing calls for its reintroduction (see Chapter 4).

The coca leaf was not burned but chewed by Peruvian Indians and was regarded by the Incas as a symbol of divinity. The Spanish conquistadores, however, regarded coca chewing as a vice, and, unlike tobacco, this habit was never introduced into European society. When the active ingredient cocaine was isolated as a pure chemical by the German chemist Albert Niemann in 1860, however, the drug suddenly became popular because of its medicinal properties. It was the first effective local anaesthetic to be used in delicate surgery on the eye and in dentistry. For a decade or more cocaine was used for a variety of medical conditions, and was famously championed by Sigmund Freud. Cocaine was said to be effective in treating a variety of nervous complaints and also began to be used recreationally. The original Coca-Cola® contained cocaine as an infusion of coca leaves, and a range of 'coca wine' preparations became available as patent medicines; lozenges containing cocaine were even marketed by the E. Merck Company to impart a 'silvery quality' to the singing voice. Ironically, one of the medical uses was in the treatment of opium addiction – a condition that was beginning to be recognized in the late nineteenth century. The powerful addictive properties of cocaine soon became apparent, however, and both medical and non-medical use fell almost completely out of favour until the modern revival of cocaine as a recreational drug in the late twentieth century.

Opium, the dried resin of the poppy plant, is another example of an ancient medicine that also served recreational purposes throughout history. Opium is one of the oldest effective painkillers, and figures prominently in both Eastern and Western herbal medicine. In Britain opium was imported in large quantities throughout the nineteenth century and enjoyed unrestricted medical and non-medical use. The impoverished labourer could buy a sample of raw opium from the corner shop and enjoy an evening of oblivion; the middle-class matron

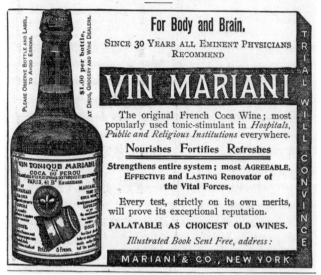

5. Cocaine-containing medicines were freely sold in the early twentieth century as remedies for a variety of ills. This advert promotes one of the many different coca wines that were recommended as 'tonic-stimulants'.

would use the more refined laudanum – an alcoholic extract of opium, diluted in water and consumed to while away the dull afternoons. Opium, and later the pure compound morphine, formed the base for hundreds of different medicines. Opium consumption rose to new heights in the latter part of the nineteenth century, and the invention of the hypodermic syringe in 1850 allowed morphine and the more powerful synthetic derivative heroin to be administered directly into the blood. There were no restrictions on opium use in England until 1868, when the first Pharmacy Act became law. It was only then that addiction was recognized as a problem on both sides of the Atlantic. By 1900 it was estimated that one in 500 of the US population was addicted to opium and strict regulation of supply soon followed – with only mixed success.

Opium in nineteenth-century Britain

'The opium preparations on sale and stocked by chemist's shops were numerous. There were opium pills (or soap and opium, and lead and opium pills), opiate lozenges, compound powder of opium, opiate confection, opiate plaster, opium enema, opium linament, vinegar of opium and wine of opium. There was a famous tincture of opium (opium dissolved in alcohol), known as laudanum, which had widespread popular sale, and the camphorated tincture, or paregoric. The dried capsules of the poppy were used, as were poppy fomentation, syrup of white poppy and extract of poppy. There were nationally famous and long established preparations like Dover's Powder, that mixture of ipecacuanha and powdered opium originally prescribed for gout by Dr Thomas Dover. . . . An expanding variety of commercial preparations began to come on the market at mid-century. They were typified by the chlorodynes – Collis Browne's, Towle's and Freeman's. The children's opiates like Godfrey's Cordial and Dalby's Carminative were long established [and used by working mothers to keep their children quiet while they went out to work]. They were everywhere to be bought. There were local preparations, too, like Kendal Black Drop, popularly supposed to be four times the strength of laudanum – and well known outside its locality because Coleridge used it. Poppy head tea in the Fens, 'sleepy beer' in the Crickhowell area, Nepenthe, Owbridge's Lung Tonic, Battley's sedative solution – popular remedies, patent medicines and the opium preparations of the textbooks were all available.'

Berridge and Edwards (1981)

The twentieth century saw the first entirely synthetic drugs that alter consciousness. The first of these were the amphetamines. d-Amphetamine (dexedrine) was first synthesized in the early twentieth century and used because of its ability to constrict blood vessels. Given by drops or inhaler, it helped to ease nasal congestion. During the Second World War dexedrine took on a new role as a stimulant that was used to keep military personnel alert and awake for long periods – for example, bomber crews on long flying missions. More potent forms of amphetamine, for example, methamphetamine ('Speed'), and new forms of administering this drug by smoking continue to be widely abused. The remarkable story of d-LSD was another later example of the synthesis of a powerful mind-altering chemical – in this case entirely by accident.

The discovery of LSD accompanied the rediscovery of other plant-derived hallucinogens – mescaline from the Mexican peyote cactus, and psilocybin from the Mexican 'Magic Mushroom' teonanactl. Both had featured prominently in ancient religious rites. These hallucinogens were joined by the ultimate synthetic recreational drug 'Ecstasy' in the later twentieth century – a compound that combines the stimulant properties of dexedrine with mild mescaline-like hallucinogenic properties.

Throughout history the medical and non-medical uses of drugs have been closely interrelated. Thus, morphine has always been one of the most important drugs in the pharmacopoeia – but also one of the most dangerous drugs of abuse (see Chapter 4). In the early years of the new millennium there is a campaign to reintroduce cannabis into Western medicine, whereas its recreational use continues to be banned in most countries. When ether was first introduced as an anaesthetic, it was fashionable for gentlemen in London clubs to amuse themselves by holding 'ether parties', and inhaling solvents remains one of the cheapest and most widely abused means of intoxication. The history of cocaine provides another example of a compound that was initially held

The discovery of d-LSD

The Swiss chemist Albert Hoffmann first synthesized d-lysergic acid diethylamide (d-LSD) in 1938 as one of a series of chemicals related to ergotamine, a drug isolated from a fungus that sometimes grew on crops of rye. Five years later he resynthesized the compound, and unwittingly received a minute dose of this powerful hallucinogen – perhaps through his skin. He describes what happened next:

'How dull would life be, if one of its dominating factors, what we call accident or chance were missing, and if we would never become surprised. I was very surprised, when in the afternoon of 16 April 1943, after I had repeated the synthesis of LSD, I entered suddenly into a kind of dreamworld. The surroundings had changed in a strange way, and had become luminous, more expressive. I felt uneasy and went home, where I wanted to rest. Lying on the couch with closed eyes, because I experienced daylight as unpleasantly glaring, I perceived an uninterrupted stream of fantastic pictures, with an intense kaleidoscopic play of colors. After some hours this strange but not unpleasant condition faded away.'

Hoffmann (1994)

in high esteem as a cure-all medicine and only later took on its present demonic form. The use of this and other 'recreational drugs' will be revisited in Chapter 4.

During the twentieth century there were dramatic increases in both the medical and the recreational use of drugs. In the medical field breakthroughs occurred in our ability to control life-threatening illnesses, and for the first time drugs were allowed for us to take control of our own reproduction. The increased use of recreational drugs occurred in response both to poverty and deprivation in some communities, and to affluence in others. Supplying and marketing both legal and illegal drugs became a major worldwide industry, accounting for a significant proportion of all economic activity. The following chapters will attempt to summarize some of these changes, and to explain our greatly improved scientific understanding of how drugs work.

Chapter 2
How drugs work

Drugs are chemicals: a series of atoms bonded together to form a molecule. They can be of natural origin – extracted from plants, animals, or microbes. For example, many antibiotics used in the treatment of infectious diseases are chemicals synthesized by one micro-organism to protect itself against others. The powerful anti-cancer drug taxol is extracted from the leaves of the yew tree. But in the twenty-first century most drugs are man-made chemicals designed to act on some particular biochemical target.

For practical reasons drugs are usually relatively small molecules, containing 10–100 atoms. Larger molecules, such as proteins (2,000–20,000 atoms), are not easily absorbed into the body and tend to be rapidly degraded on entry. Medicines contain the active drug molecule along with various other inactive ingredients, sugars, starches, or oils to make a tablet or other preparation. The amount of active drug is usually minute, measured in a few thousandths of a gram; it would be impractical to handle and manufacture tablets unless they contained the various inert filler materials.

Most medicines are taken by mouth in tablet or capsule form, but some are given as liquids (easier for children or old people to swallow), or by other routes of delivery. When medicines are given by mouth, they are

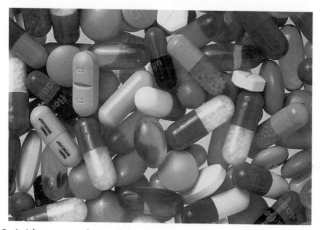

6. A rich armoury of powerful medicines is available to the modern physician.

gradually absorbed into the bloodstream from the stomach and gut. This is a relatively slow process – but this is not a drawback if the medicine is being used to treat a long-term disease, where a sustained delivery of drug is needed. The ideal medicine for such diseases is taken by mouth once a day – but this requires that there is a steady absorption from the gut and that the active drug is not degraded too rapidly in the body. Absorption from the gut need not involve swallowing the drug – another method is to administer the drug incorporated into a waxy suppository inserted into the rectum. This too gives a slow and sustained absorption of the active material and is a popular method of drug delivery in several European countries. I will never forget the occasion when my wife developed a sore throat in Paris some years ago and went to a pharmacy to obtain some medicine. She emerged with some strange-looking waxy lozenges, which she was about to swallow before our friends told her the correct means of administration! In Anglo-Saxon countries we are more prudish and the rectal suppository has never been popular.

Some drugs require more rapid delivery – for example, an antibiotic given to treat a severe infection or an anaesthetic administered for a surgical operation. In such cases a drug solution can be injected directly into the blood via a vein. Intravenous injection is also a route favoured by drug addicts to deliver, for example, heroin – this route provides almost instant delivery of the drug to the brain, giving the maximum 'high'. Other drugs are unstable in the gut and thus cannot be delivered by mouth and must be given by injection – often into muscle or just under the skin (for example, insulin for diabetes). Recreational drug-users and addicts favour smoking as a means of rapid delivery of drugs such as nicotine (tobacco smoke), cannabis, cocaine, heroin, or amphetamines. Many drugs are rapidly absorbed into the blood vessels present in the large internal surface area of the lungs. The cigarette-smoker can obtain a pulse of nicotine to the brain within seconds of lighting up – and can then adjust the delivery of nicotine very precisely by controlling the frequency of puffs and the depth of inhalation. Because of the rapid delivery offered by this route, many anaesthetics are delivered by inhalation; as with the cigarette-smoker, the anaesthetist can control the level of anaesthesia very precisely by varying the rate of drug delivery. Some drugs are delivered locally to the site in the body at which they are needed – thus avoiding exposure of the whole body to what might be an undesirably large dose of the drug. For example, an aerosol of drug-containing fluid droplets is inhaled into the lung to control the symptoms of asthma; ointments are rubbed into the skin for pain relief; or medicines are given directly to the eye in the form of drops. Drugs used to treat disorders of the brain have to have special properties because the brain is insulated from the bloodstream by a specialized 'blood–brain barrier', which protects the brain from the possibly harmful effects of chemicals absorbed in the diet. Only small and relatively fat-soluble drug molecules are able to penetrate this barrier.

There have been several modern improvements in drug delivery systems. Special tablets can be designed that dissolve only slowly in the

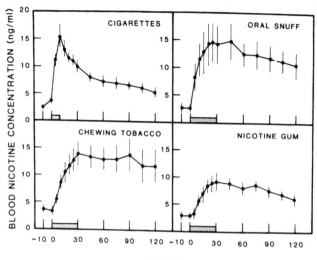

7. Absorption of nicotine via different routes. Drugs are absorbed into the bloodstream at different rates according to the route of administration. In the case of nicotine, smoking is the fastest means of delivering the drug, which is rapidly absorbed by the large surface area of the lungs.

gut – providing an extended period of drug absorption. In this way it has been possible, for example, to develop a once-a-day preparation of morphine for pain relief – a considerable achievement for a drug that is inactivated quite rapidly and normally has to be given every four hours. Another advance has been the development of adhesive skin patches that contain an active drug and allow its prolonged absorption through the skin. This, for example, is a widely used means of delivering oestrogen as hormone replacement therapy for post-menopausal women. A remarkable system has been developed that delivers powdered drugs or vaccines into the skin using a high powered jet of gas – allowing needle-less injections.

Drug receptors

Whatever route of delivery is used, either the drug molecule must end up in the bloodstream – from which it can exit freely into virtually any organ of the body (apart from the brain) – or the drug must be delivered locally to the target organ. In the target organ, the drug is recognized by 'receptors'. These are large molecules, usually proteins, to which the drug binds tightly and with a high degree of specificity. Small changes in the chemistry of the drug molecule may yield analogues that are unable to bind and are consequently inactive. The drug often binds to a site in the protein normally occupied by some naturally occurring small molecule. Occupation of this site by the drug molecule then either mimics the effect normally elicited by that natural chemical (for drugs known as 'agonists') or blocks it ('antagonists'). For example, there are so-called beta-receptors in the heart, which recognize the cardiac stimulant hormone adrenaline. Adrenaline itself (the agonist) can be used in medical emergencies to stimulate the failing heart, but synthetic drugs called beta-blockers, which act as antagonists at the cardiac beta-receptors, are also valuable medicines, which are used to treat heart disease and high blood pressure (see Chapter 3).

Many drugs act on receptor protein molecules that normally function in cell signalling mechanisms. These proteins are located at the cell surface in various tissues (muscle, nerve, gut, brain, and so on). They may recognize and be activated by hormones carried in the bloodstream. For example, adrenaline (epinephrine) is secreted into the blood at times of stress and prepares the body for 'fight or flight'. It acts as a trigger for receptors present in many different parts of the body. Adrenaline stimulates the heart to pump more blood, mobilizes energy reserves in muscle, increases the rate of breathing, and in animals with fur it causes the individual hairs to rise – making the animal look bigger and more ferocious. Receptors on nerve cells recognize and respond to the many other different chemical messenger molecules used for communication between such cells in the brain. Under normal conditions, the binding of the natural signal molecule activates such receptor proteins. This leads to a subtle change in the shape of the protein, which may trigger changes in the permeability of the cell to sodium, potassium, calcium, or other inorganic ions, thus altering its excitability. Alternatively, the activated receptor may trigger the synthesis of other internal signalling molecules within the cell, the so-called second messengers that alter the cell's metabolism. Several hundred such cell surface receptor proteins are known – and more are being discovered, as we understand more about the human genome. A typical receptor protein consists of 400–500 amino-acid residues. It is folded and inserted into the cell membrane in such a way that there are seven regions of the protein within the membrane and some regions protruding on both external and internal surfaces. Detailed knowledge of the molecular architecture of such receptors is helping us to understand better how they work, and in future may help in the design of drug molecules to fit the receptor even more precisely.

Other proteins located at the surface of the cell can also be drug targets. A large family of proteins function as gatekeepers, regulating the levels of chemicals in the cell, particularly the components of the salty solution in which all living cells are bathed. These include sodium, potassium, calcium, chloride, and other inorganic salts. The gatekeeper proteins form minute channels in the cell membrane through which such chemicals can enter or exit living cells – and by changes in the protein's shape these channels can be opened or closed according to need. Such channels are particularly important in nerve cells and in muscle, which rely on an imbalance between salts inside and outside the cell to generate the minute pulses of electricity by which nerve signals are transmitted or which cause muscles to contract. These channels offer a rich variety of drug targets. The ancient remedy digitalis, extracted from the foxglove plant, for example, acts by blocking sodium channels in heart muscle, preventing potentially dangerous overactivity. Other cell surface proteins act as 'pumps' that transport chemicals from one side of the cell membrane to the other – usually from the outside to the inside. They have a number of functions – for example, in delivering glucose or other nutrients to the cell, or in removing biologically active chemicals from the cell surface. The antidepressant drug Prozac, for example, acts by blocking a pump whose function is to remove the chemical messenger molecule serotonin after its release from activated nerve cells. Blocking this pump has the effect of prolonging the actions of serotonin in the brain – and this appears to underlie its antidepressant properties (see Chapter 3).

Drugs may act on biochemical targets within the cell as well as at the cell surface. Some drugs bind directly to DNA in the nucleus and interfere with the normal process of reading DNA sequences into proteins, thereby inhibiting cell division and growth. This can be particularly important in some drugs used to control the growth of cancer cells. Other targets inside the cell include enzymes. Enzymes are proteins that have the special function of acting as catalysts to promote particular chemical reactions that are involved in the breakdown of foodstuffs to produce energy, or in the synthesis of one or other of the complex chemicals that make up the body. Such chemical syntheses often involve a complex series of reactions and a number of different enzymes. Blocking the action of one enzyme with a drug can, however, block the whole pathway. This strategy has yielded many very important medical drugs. For example, many antibiotics act by blocking the synthesis of key components of the bacterial cell wall, thus preventing further bacterial multiplication; cholesterol-lowering drugs inhibit an enzyme involved in cholesterol synthesis. Enzyme proteins contain an 'active site' that normally binds the chemical substrate of the enzyme. Inhibitor drugs usually bind to the same site and prevent the enzyme from functioning. Enzymes are often soluble proteins present in the cell sap within living cells. For technical reasons, this makes it easier to obtain precise information on their three-dimensional molecular structure – and this in turn assists in the application of computer-aided molecular modelling techniques to design drugs that target that particular enzyme and 'dock' into its active site.

The science of 'molecular pharmacology', which aims to study the details of how small drug molecules interact with their large protein targets, advanced greatly during the last decades of the twentieth century. This was largely due to powerful new technology that allows scientists to manipulate DNA molecules. The long thread-like DNA molecules carry the information needed to specify proteins encoded in the sequence of the four bases of which they are composed – Adenine, Thymine, Cytosine, and Guanine. The DNA for an individual gene consists of a sequence of several thousand bases that specifies the sequence of the twenty different amino-acid building blocks that are linked together to form a protein, containing on average 500–1,000 amino acids. It is now possible to isolate the DNA encoding for a particular protein and insert this into an immortalized tissue culture cell. The resulting newly created cells will grow and divide and will contain the protein of interest. Molecular pharmacologists can thus study human drug receptors under laboratory conditions – and can use these model systems to discover new drugs that target that particular receptor. This technology can be applied both to cell surface receptor proteins and to enzymes. For enzymes it is also possible to insert the human gene into a bacterium, which will then make the human enzyme. It is easy to grow large quantities of bacteria, so in this way it is possible to produce large amounts of human enzyme protein that can later be extracted and purified. Enzyme proteins that may be present normally only in minute amounts in the body can thus be produced in large quantities for laboratory studies and for use in screening new drugs. The new era of molecular pharmacology allows scientists to study human drug receptors in a way that was not possible before. Previous studies of drug receptors have relied on using indirect tests of receptor function – in which the receptor was a 'black box' of unknown biochemical composition. Prior to the molecular pharmacology era, studying the actions of drugs on receptors usually also involved using receptors in animal tissues. Although human drug receptors and those found in laboratory animals (rats and mice) are usually very similar, there can be important species differences.

Measuring the effects of drugs

Although molecular techniques can tell us a great deal about the way in which drug molecules interact with their receptors, other methods are needed to assess the effects of drugs in the body. Some of the biological effects of drugs can be studied in human or animal cells grown in tissue culture in the laboratory. Thus, the actions of drugs on the electrical activity of brain cells can be examined by using minute needle-like electrodes to record such activity directly from individual nerve cells growing in tissue culture. Alternatively, heart muscle cells in tissue culture can be used to examine the effects of drugs on the excitability of the heart. The effectiveness of new antibiotics in killing bacteria or other micro-organisms can also readily be assessed in the test tube or Petri dish. A whole era of pharmacology relied on the use of isolated animal organs after removal from the body (for example, heart, muscle, segments of gut), which continue to contract for some time after removal if incubated in oxygenated warm saline solution. Drugs can then be added to the 'organ bath' and their effects studied by measuring the resulting changes in muscle contraction or heart beat.

Eventually, however, we want to know what effects drugs have on the whole organism. If we want to study the effects of drugs on blood pressure, we cannot expect to do this just by examining their effects on cells in tissue culture or on isolated organs; we need to measure blood pressure in human or animal subjects. If we are interested in testing new drugs to treat epileptic seizures, we need to use animal models in which epileptic seizures can be simulated by various means. In the final analysis, we need to give the drugs to human patients suffering from epilepsy to see if they are effective. However, it would be unethical to give new drugs of unknown toxicity to human subjects in the first instance, so animal experiments still inevitably play a crucial role in studying the effects of drugs. The advent of molecular techniques that allow the initial screening of new compounds to be carried out with human cells in the laboratory means that the numbers of animals needed for drug research has gone down markedly in recent years. A large range of different animal models exists for studying the effects of various categories of drugs. In cases where the medical end point is clearly defined and the biological mechanisms well understood – for example, in lowering blood pressure, reducing blood cholesterol, reducing inflammation, or fighting infectious diseases – the animal models can often provide a fairly precise replica of the human disease. In other illnesses, however, particularly in such mental disorders as depression, anxiety, or schizophrenia, there is much less understanding of the biological basis of the illness. Animal models in these instances are often complex behavioural tests, chosen because existing drugs that are known to be effective in these diseases have some clear effect.

Whatever test system is used, whether it is a simple biochemical measurement of drug/receptor binding in the test tube or the recording of a complex physiological or behavioural response in the whole animal, a key issue is to determine the effective drug dose. The drug concentration needed to occupy the receptor, and hence to produce a response, is determined by the affinity of the drug for the target receptor. If the affinity is high, only low concentrations of the drug will be needed, and only very low doses will be needed to elicit the desired response in the whole animal. To find out what the effective concentration is in the drug/receptor assay, or what dose is needed in the whole animal or person, a wide range of different drug concentrations or doses needs to be tested. The results can be presented as a graph showing the drug response with increasing doses – the so-called dose-response curve. As the range of effective drug concentrations often spans a range of more than a thousandfold, the drug concentration is usually depicted on a log scale (see Figure 8). The

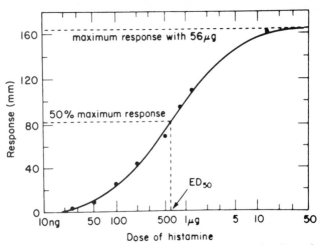

8. Typical 'Dose-response curve'. Pharmacologists measure the effects of increasing doses of drug to find the maximum response and the 'effective dose 50' or 'ED50', which causes half of the maximum response. In this instance the contraction of a piece of guinea pig small intestine was measured in response to increasing doses of histamine.

dose-response curve is useful, as it allows one to compare the potencies of a range of different drugs that act on the same receptor. Although the actions of drugs reflect their ability to occupy their particular receptor targets, the dose-response curve generated in the test tube or tissue culture model is not always reflected in the whole animal. When drugs are administered, they may not reach their desired targets, or they may be inactivated very rapidly. Drugs that target receptors in the brain may not be able to penetrate the blood–brain barrier. Thus, although the drug may have a high affinity for the right receptor, it may be quite inactive in the whole animal or person.

Finding the most suitable dose is one of the most difficult questions in using drugs to treat medical conditions. Virtually all drugs will produce undesirable side effects if too high a dose is given. These side effects can range from minor discomforts to life-threatening damage to vital organs – often gut, liver, or kidney. Even aspirin, a drug commonly believed to be safe, can cause dangerous irritation and bleeding in the stomach and intestine. Thousands of patients die each year from gastric bleeding caused by aspirin and the more powerful newer aspirin-like drugs. Herbal medicines are not exempt: in Belgium recently a number of patients suffered severe kidney damage caused by the Chinese herb *Aristolochia fangchi*, and several patients had to undergo kidney transplant operations. For most drugs there is an optimum range of doses that produces the maximum medical benefit without adverse side effects. The separation between the dose range in which the desirable medical benefits are seen, and the higher dose range at which adverse effects emerge, is known as the 'therapeutic window'. Obviously, it is desirable that this window should be as big as possible, but it is not always possible to achieve this. The adverse side effects may be caused by overstimulation of the same receptor mechanism that underlies the therapeutic effects. Thus, for example, morphine is widely used in treating severe pain, but the therapeutic window is relatively small and, at higher doses, nausea and vomiting, confusion, respiratory depression, and constipation are all common side effects, and these are all mediated by the same opiate receptor mechanism that mediates pain relief. Similarly, one of the problems encountered in the medical use of cannabis is that there is only a narrow therapeutic window between the doses that yield beneficial medical effects and the doses that cause intoxication. Although the intoxicant effects are what the recreational user wants from the drug, these effects are usually unwanted and can be frightening to the elderly patient not familiar with the drug. The therapeutic-window concept applies equally importantly to the recreational use of drugs. Even the experienced heroin or cocaine user sometimes gets it wrong and ends up administering a lethal overdose.

Finding the most suitable therapeutic dose for a new drug, and determining the size of the therapeutic window, may be among the most difficult parts of any drug development. Because individual human

differ in size and in the way in which they inactivate drug
ules, it may not be possible to define a dose that will be optimum
for all patients, and it may be necessary to find this out by trial and error.
The optimum dose may be different for men and women, who
sometimes inactivate drugs differently; children and old people are also
less able to inactivate drugs quickly, so they may need smaller doses
than healthy adults.

How drugs are inactivated in the body

As far as the body is concerned, drugs, whether natural or man-made,
are foreign substances and a series of complex defences have evolved to
inactivate and eliminate such materials. In the natural environment
humans and other animals encounter a wide range of chemicals in their
diet, many of which can have biological effects. It is clearly undesirable
that such potentially dangerous chemicals should be allowed to
accumulate – they must be detoxified and eliminated. Man-made drugs
can also be inactivated and eliminated by these mechanisms, and this
poses a problem for the pharmacologist. If the drug is inactivated and
eliminated too rapidly, the drug will be effective for only a short period
of time, and repeat dosing may be needed. In some instances – for
example, in the use of morphine to control severe pain – the drug may
need to be taken every few hours. The ideal for the long-term treatment
of chronic illnesses is obviously a medicine that needs to be taken only
once a day.

Some drugs will be excreted unchanged in the urine. The kidney has a
number of specialized pump mechanisms that remove substances
actively from the blood and pass them out in the urine – these
mechanisms apply particularly to drugs that have some acidic or
alkaline character that can be recognized by these kidney mechanisms.
Fat-soluble drugs may be removed quite rapidly from the circulation, as
they tend to become concentrated in fat stores in the body. Such drugs
may persist for long periods in the fat stores and gradually leak out into

circulation and become excreted. While dissolved in the fat, the drugs are not biologically active, as they do not have access to their receptors. Cannabis and some of its metabolites, for example, persist in the fat stores of the body for several weeks after a single dose. Because minute amounts leak out of the fat stores and are excreted in urine, the unfortunate recreational user can yield a urine-positive cannabis drug test more than one week after a single exposure to the drug.

By far the most important means of inactivating drugs is by metabolism – using enzymes to convert them to harmless products, which can then be eliminated from the body. Much of this drug metabolism takes place in the liver, which is rich in a wide range of different drug-metabolizing enzymes. The liver is strategically placed. As it receives all of the blood coming from the gut before it enters the general circulation, it can eliminate toxic chemicals absorbed from the diet before they can do too much harm. Drug molecules are attacked by one or more of the liver enzymes and converted into inactive by-products that are then excreted, either in the bile from the liver, discharged into the gut and eventually eliminated in the faeces, or by the kidney into the urine. The drug-metabolizing enzymes in the liver, called cytochrome-p450s, comprise a large family of some fifty or more related enzymes, which have evolved in a remarkable way; they can deal with essentially any foreign chemical – including man-made drugs that by definition are never normally encountered in nature. Many drugs are given repeatedly for long periods of time and the liver and kidney are called upon every day to eliminate these foreign chemicals. These organs are also exposed to high concentrations of the drugs as they are first absorbed from the gut and channelled through the liver, and the drug or its metabolite may be concentrated in the kidney for excretion in the urine. It is not surprising, therefore, that the liver and the kidney are the organs that are most vulnerable to drug-induced damage. This can sometimes be serious and even life threatening. The metabolism of drugs in the liver can also sometimes produce toxic metabolites that make matters worse – as in the case of the relatively harmless drug paracetamol, which can be degraded to form a liver-damaging metabolite.

One way of minimizing these risks is to develop and use more and more potent drugs, so that the amount of foreign chemical that needs to be given is reduced. In the older generation of medical drugs it was not uncommon to need doses of 1 gram or more each day, whereas with many modern drugs the doses needed are 100–1,000 times lower.

The efficiency of the various mechanisms for drug metabolism and elimination poses a challenge to the pharmacologist, because these processes limit the duration of action of drugs. Some drugs may be well absorbed from the gut, but may suffer extensive metabolic degradation in the liver before they have a chance to enter the general circulation and exert their beneficial effects. An additional problem that is often encountered is that different drugs may compete for the same liver enzymes. In this case, their duration of action and peak blood levels may be altered when given together, often with adverse consequences. Such drug interactions are common, particularly in elderly patients, who tend to be taking several different medicines every day. Prolonged regimes of drug treatment can cause another problem. If the same drug is taken repeatedly, it may lead to a large increase in the liver enzyme(s) involved in its metabolism; this means that the drug will tend to become less and less effective over time – a phenomenon known as 'tolerance'. Drug interactions may also be seen in such instances: if drug A leads to a large increase in liver enzyme activity, it may accelerate the disposal of drug B if this is metabolized by the same enzyme(s). Extracts of St John's Wort have become popular as a natural antidepressant, for example, but it has become apparent that the herbal medicine causes increases in a number of liver enzymes and this can alter the effectiveness of several prescription drugs – notably the oral contraceptives and drugs used to treat AIDS.

We are also becoming increasingly aware of genetic factors that alter drug responsiveness in some individuals. For example, 6 per cent of the Caucasian population lack the genes encoding one of the cytochrome p450 drug-metabolizing enzymes known as CYP2D6. This enzyme is importantly involved in the metabolism of about a quarter of all prescription drugs. Such individuals have a serious impairment in their ability to detoxify and eliminate these drugs and may thus overreact when treated with normal therapeutic doses. The study of genetic factors that determine drug responses is a new subject called 'pharmacogenomics'.

Effects of long-term drug administration

Many drugs are used to treat chronic medical conditions and increasingly drugs are given prophylactically to prevent the development of a medical condition – as, for example, with the cholesterol-lowering agents (see Chapter 3). Such long-term dosage regimes may carry risks. As pointed out above, it is not uncommon for the drugs to become less effective with time, because they cause an increase in liver-metabolizing enzymes. This is less likely to occur with modern highly potent drugs, as the increase in liver enzymes is usually seen only in response to relatively high doses of drug, which swamp the liver's capacity to metabolize them. There are, however, other mechanisms that can lead to the development of drug tolerance. The use of morphine and related drugs as painkillers, for example, is complicated by the fact that most patients develop tolerance to the drug and require increasing doses – sometimes the drug becomes virtually ineffective even when given in very large doses. A tolerant patient can take as much as 1 gram of morphine a day – a dose that would prove lethal to a drug-naïve subject. In this case, the mechanisms responsible for the development of tolerance are not understood, but the phenomenon is nevertheless very real. Other drugs that act on the central nervous system also exhibit tolerance – and some also lead to the development of addiction, or 'substance dependence', as it is now more correctly called (see Chapter 4).

Our understanding of how drugs work increased greatly during the twentieth century. This ushered in an era of rational drug discovery, in which new drugs are made to target the particular biochemical mechanisms that are believed to be defective in individual diseases. The twenty-first century will see this approach extended, as we become able to design drugs that will best suit the individual patient.

Chapter 3
Drugs as medicines

The physician in the twenty-first century has an impressive range of powerful medicines at his or her command. It is possible to treat a number of hitherto untreatable conditions with effective medicines, and these often represent the most cost-effective way of managing illness by comparison with costly surgery or hospital care. Spending on drugs represents an average of around 10 per cent of the total health budget in most developed countries, and this is likely to rise still further as the next generation of 'biologicals' becomes available.

Medicines include the ever-popular herbal remedies, a variety of other natural products, and a host of man-made chemicals. A new generation of biological products is becoming increasingly important – they include human proteins that are used to replace their defective counterparts in some human diseases, and an increasing number of antibodies. These are proteins that are normally formed by the immune system as part of the body's defence against infections or invasion by other foreign bodies. The modern generation of 'monoclonal antibodies', however, are made in the laboratory and designed to target and inactivate various key proteins known to be involved in the processes underlying various diseases. The powerful techniques of molecular biology make it possible to synthesize such human antibodies and other human proteins on a large scale and to use them as medicines. Most human proteins exist in only tiny amounts in the body, and hitherto the only way of obtaining them in any quantity was to purify them from blood or from human or animal tissues. For example, until recently most diabetic patients were treated with insulin purified from pig pancreas, but this is now largely replaced by the man-made human hormone. Biological products are generally large proteins that cannot be absorbed when given by mouth – they have to be given by injection. Sometimes this may be needed several times a day (for example, insulin) but in other cases treatment once a week or once a month in the doctor's surgery may be sufficient.

Some medicines that are regarded as particularly safe to use can be obtained 'over the counter' in any pharmacy. These include such widely used drugs as the painkillers aspirin and paracetamol and a large number of medicines for coughs, colds, and other minor ailments. Such medicines are often based on traditional remedies and include a number of mildly active ingredients, together with sugars and flavouring to help make the medicine go down! Most new medical drugs, however, start life as prescription medicines. There is not enough experience of the possible hazards of a new medicine to make it safe to sell 'over the counter' and the doctor controls the use of such medicines by writing a prescription and carefully monitoring the patient's response. After many years of experience of the widespread use of a new prescription medicine, it may become clear that the compound is relatively safe to use – and it may then be sold 'over the counter'. In the 1990s, for example, a number of the powerful drugs used to treat stomach ulcers became available in this way – having first been available only as prescription drugs for nearly twenty years. On the other hand, with some drugs there will always be a risk to the patient if the dose is not right, or there may be the potential for diverting the medical drug to recreational use. It is unlikely, for example, that such drugs as antibiotics or those used to treat heart conditions will be made into 'over-the-counter' products; and, although morphine was available 'over the counter' in Victorian times, this is not likely to happen again.

This book is not intended to be a textbook of pharmacology – and in the space available it is impossible to cover the whole range of medical drugs now available. Instead a few examples will be highlighted to illustrate some of the principles underlying the successful use of medicines in the treatment of illnesses. Large omissions from this chapter include the drug treatment of blood diseases, diabetes, and other hormonal diseases. The challenge of the drug treatment of cancer and the impact of drugs used to control human reproduction will be discussed in Chapter 6.

Fighting heart disease

In 1628 William Harvey published his famous book *De motu cordis* in which he described the pumping action of the heart. Careful studies of various animals and human demonstrations led him to the then revolutionary idea that the blood circulated around the body, propelled by the heart acting as a pump. Hitherto it had been thought that the heart pumped air to cool the blood, aided by the lungs. We now know that the 4 litres or so of blood in an average human is pumped by the heart through the lungs for oxygenation and then via the arteries to all the tissues of the body, from which it is returned to the heart through the veins. The human heart has to perform prodigious mechanical feats – pumping the relatively viscous blood at quite high pressure through the millions of tiny capillary vessels in the tissues, and beating regularly for an entire lifetime. Its job is made more difficult in many people as they grow older because they develop abnormally high blood pressure. This is caused by the narrowing of blood vessels with age, making it more difficult for the heart to force the blood through them at normal pressure. These changes can be made worse by many different causes, of which obesity, too salty a diet, and smoking are some of the commonest. The high fat content of most Western diets tends to promote high blood levels of the insoluble fatty material cholesterol and this leads to the laying-down of deposits of cholesterol in the lining of the arteries. This in turn constricts the arteries and tends to lead to raised blood pressure. The cholesterol deposits are particularly dangerous when they affect the coronary arteries, the blood vessels within the heart muscle itself that supply it with oxygen and nutrients. The combination of raised blood pressure, which puts a greater burden on the heart as a pump, and partial blockade of the coronary arteries can lead to sudden heart failure, when one or more of the coronary vessels becomes entirely blocked. The outcome can be death or recovery with a damaged heart, resulting in prolonged or permanent impairment. Coronary heart disease is one of the most common diseases in the Western world and it remains one of the leading causes of death. High blood pressure and constricted arteries to the brain can also lead to stroke – a sudden interruption of the blood supply to vital areas of the brain. This too can lead to death or serious disability. Nevertheless, the advent of powerful new medicines is beginning to change these statistics and such changes will continue during the initial decades of the twenty-first century, as the new treatments begin to show their long-term beneficial effects. The successful treatment of high blood pressure, heart disease, and abnormally high cholesterol were major achievements for pharmacology in the latter half of the twentieth century.

The drugs used to treat high blood pressure come in many different varieties. Among the earliest to be developed were 'water pills' (diuretics), which promote urine production in the kidney. By removing some of the water content of the blood in this way, the drugs reduce the volume of circulating blood and consequently lower blood pressure. There are more than two dozen different diuretic drugs available and they continue to be widely used as a cheap and moderately effective first line of attack on the problem.

The first modern breakthrough in the field came from one of the greatest drug discoverers of the twentieth century, James (now Sir James) Black, in the 1960s. At that time he was working for the pharmaceutical company ICI and he discovered the first of the 'beta-blockers'. These drugs target and block the beta-receptors that are present in the heart. These receptors respond to adrenaline secreted into the blood in conditions of stress from the adrenal gland, and to noradrenaline, a chemical messenger secreted by the nerve fibres that innervate and control the heart. In either case, stimulation of the beta-receptor causes the heart to increase its rate of contraction and also the strength of each beat. This consequently tends to raise blood pressure. The beta-blockers counteract these effects by preventing the actions of adrenaline and noradrenaline, and consequently they lower blood pressure. In addition, by reducing the amount of work the heart has to do, they are also beneficial in patients suffering from heart failure, a gradual loss of heart function that is common in the elderly. The beta-blockers are widely used as a first line of treatment for high blood pressure and heart disease.

Another important advance was the discovery of 'calcium channel blockers'. These drugs act on the muscle that lines the arteries and controls the extent to which the arteries are constricted or relaxed. Obviously it is harder to pump blood through arteries that are constricted, so contraction of the muscle tends to raise blood pressure. An inward movement of the inorganic salt calcium into the cell triggers the contraction of the muscle cells lining the blood vessels, and these drugs act by partially blocking these channels. Consequently they tend to cause the arteries to relax and offer less resistance to blood flow – thus lowering blood pressure. There are many different drugs in this class and they have proved very successful. Tthe calcium antagonists represent one of the top ten classes of prescription drugs in terms of commercial value, with worldwide sale of nearly $10 billion in 1999 (Table 1). (Note that this does not mean that beta-blockers are not equally widely used, but the beta-blockers are older drugs whose patents have expired – consequently they are now relatively cheap medicines; see Chapter 5 below.)

A completely different mechanism underlies the therapeutic effects of yet another class of drugs for treating high blood pressure and heart failure, the 'ACE inhibitors'. One of the most powerful triggers for the contraction of the artery muscles is the hormone angiotensin. It plays a key role in regulating blood pressure and fluid balance in the body. In addition to stimulating the arteries to constrict, angiotensin also acts on the kidneys to suppress urine production, and acts on the brain to stimulate thirst and drinking behaviour. Angiotensin is generated in the blood from an inactive precursor called renin. The conversion requires an enzyme known as Angiotensin Converting Enzyme (ACE). The idea of using ACE inhibitors to lower blood pressure arose from a discovery in the 1960s by the Brazilian scientist Sergio Ferreira. He observed that the venom of the Brazilian viper caused a profound drop in blood pressure in animals, and tracked this down to a compound in the venom that inhibited this enzyme. Scientists in the American pharmaceutical companies Squibb and later Merck used these discoveries to develop synthetic drugs that act in the same way. The ACE inhibitors have proved remarkably effective and safe to use, and, like the beta-blockers, they are useful both to lower blood pressure and to protect the failing heart. By the end of the twentieth century there were more than a dozen different drugs in this class, with annual worldwide sales of $7.4 billion in 1999. Another way of blocking the effects of angiotensin has been to develop drugs that target the receptors in the blood vessels and kidneys on which the hormone acts, rather than preventing its production. A number of angiotensin receptor antagonists have been introduced in recent years, and have proved as effective as the ACE inhibitors – and in some patients they are preferable because of a lower incidence of side effects (Figure 9).

The last category of agents in this area is the cholesterol-lowering drugs. In the Western world, our fat-rich diet and lack of exercise tend to lead to abnormally high blood levels of the fatty substance cholesterol, which tends to accumulate in deposits on the lining of blood vessels, partially blocking them. This in turn increases the risk of high blood pressure, heart failure, and stroke. Less than half of the

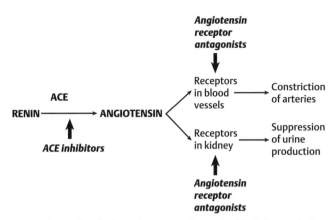

9. How drugs affect biological processes. Drugs that block the synthesis or actions of angiotensin have proved very valuable in treating high blood pressure and heart disease.

cholesterol in the blood originates from the diet; the rest is synthesized in the body, mainly in the liver. The cholesterol-lowering drugs, the so-called statins, block this synthesis by targeting a key enzyme in the synthetic pathway -HMG-CoA reductase. In this way it is possible by drug treatment to lower blood cholesterol by as much as 40–50 per cent. The statins were introduced only in the 1980s and their widespread use has become accepted only gradually over the years. They represent a new sort of medicine – one that is taken to prevent a disease from developing, rather than to treat existing symptoms. They do not lower blood pressure or treat the failing heart – but they prevent further cholesterol deposition in the arteries and may even lead to a regression of the deposits that already exist. There is now clear evidence that the statins save lives, particularly in those who have extremely high cholesterol levels or in patients who have already experienced one heart attack. They are among the first widely used 'preventive medicines'. To the pharmaceutical companies, the statins represent a bonanza – once a patient starts taking a statin, he or she will go on doing so for the rest of his or her life, and in Western societies perhaps as many as half of all adults have cholesterol levels that might be considered too high. No wonder that the sales of statins represent the second largest class of prescription medicines, with annual worldwide sales of $13.4 billion in 1999. A new generation of 'super-statins' due to be marketed in the early years of the new millennium promises to lower blood cholesterol even further than the first generation drugs could.

It is clear from these figures that the drug treatment of high blood pressure and heart disease is one of the biggest and most successful sectors of the pharmaceutical arena. Many innovative new classes of agents were introduced during the latter half of the twentieth century

TABLE 1. Top ten classes of prescription drugs in terms of commercial value, 1999

Drug class	Worldwide sales in 1999 ($bn.)	Global sales (%)
1. Anti-ulcers	15.8	5.3
2. Cholesterol lowering	13.4	4.5
3. Antidepressants	11.7	4.0
4. Calcium antagonists	9.9	3.3
5. Non-steroidal anti-inflammatories	7.7	2.6
6. ACE-inhibitors	7.4	2.5
7. Cephalosporins and related antibiotics	7.3	2.5
8. Non-narcotic painkillers	6.2	2.1
9. Anti-psychotics	5.1	1.7
10. Oral antidiabetics	4.8	1.6
TOTAL FOR TOP TEN	89.3	30.2

Source: IMS Health World Review (2000).

and individual patients can be treated with the most appropriate
cocktail of drugs for their particular condition.

Healing gastric ulcers

The stomach is a remarkable organ. When food enters the stomach, the
cells lining the stomach secrete a digestive fluid that contains quite a
high concentration of hydrochloric acid and is consequently highly
acidic. The gastric fluid also contains digestive enzymes, such as pepsin,
that can function in this unusually acidic environment. The acidic gastric
fluid helps to start the rapid chemical breakdown of foodstuffs, and at
the same time sterilizes the food by destroying most of the potentially
harmful micro-organisms that it may contain. But using such a strong
acid secretion carries its own hazards. The cells lining the stomach are
protected against acid-induced damage by a thick layer of mucus.
However, under some conditions this defence may be broken down, and
the resulting exposure of the tender lining of the organ to the acid
contents can lead to irritation and eventually to ulcers – painful areas of
damaged tissue. Ulcers are particularly likely to occur if too much acid is
secreted in the stomach – particularly when food is not present. Such
conditions can occur in response to stress of various kinds – and modern
life in big cities is full of stress. Excessive intake of alcohol can also
damage the protective lining of the stomach, and such intake of
alcohol is also a widespread feature of our society. Not surprisingly,
stomach ulcers are common.

Prior to the discovery of effective anti-ulcer drugs, the only treatment
for severe stomach ulcers was the surgical removal of the damaged part
of the stomach. The introduction of powerful new classes of anti-ulcer
drugs during the 1970s and 1980s, however, has effectively put the
gastric surgeons out of business.

The first breakthrough came again from Sir James Black in the 1970s,
who was working for the company then known as Smith Kline & French.

It had been known for some time that in the stomach the chemical messenger molecule histamine plays a key role in the train of events leading to gastric acid secretion. The intake of food triggers a release of histamine, which activates the acid-secreting cells. Anti-histamine drugs have been known for a long time and are widely used in treating the symptoms of inflammation and congestion in the lungs caused by hay fever and other allergies, and the pain and itch caused by insect bites or sunburn in the skin. The classical anti-histamine drugs, however, fail to block the actions of histamine in the stomach. James Black showed that this was because histamine acted on a different type of receptor in the stomach from those in skin or lung. He and his colleagues went on to develop the first effective antagonist drugs acting on the so-called histamine H_2 receptors in the stomach, and showed that these compounds were very effective in suppressing gastric acid secretion. This in turn helped to heal stomach ulcers, and the H_2 blockers became a very successful new class of prescription drugs. James Black won the Nobel Prize for Physiology and Medicine in 1988 for this and his earlier work on beta-blockers. The huge sales of one drug in particular, ranitidine (sold under the trade name Zantac®), helped to lift the British pharmaceutical company Glaxo into the world league. The patent lives of the first H_2 blockers have expired, but they continue to enjoy large sales as 'over-the-counter' medicines.

A second breakthrough soon followed in this field with the advent of a new class of drugs that act directly on the acid-secreting cells in the stomach to inhibit acid formation – the so-called proton-pump inhibitors. These drugs are even more effective than the H_2 blockers in almost completely suppressing gastric acid secretion. They consequently can help to heal gastric ulcers even more rapidly – with complete healing commonly seen after only one month of drug treatment. The first successful drug of this class was omeprazole (sold under the trade name Losec®), and it helped to change the medium-sized Swedish pharmaceutical company Astra, which discovered it, into a major player in the pharmaceutical industry. The combined annual worldwide sales of the H2 blockers and proton pump inhibitors of nearly $16 billion in 1999 make this one of the most commercially important of all the categories of prescription drugs.

These are not the only medicines that are important in the treatment of gastric ulcers. One puzzling feature of the successful treatment of ulcers with H2 blockers or proton-pump inhibitors is that after some time, when the ulcers have healed and the drug treatment stopped, patients often suffer a recurrence. Is this simply because the drugs do not remove the stress that is the underlying cause, or are there other factors? The answer came as a big surprise, in the form of a newly discovered bacterium *Helicobacter pylori*, an organism that has evolved to adapt to the harsh conditions inside the stomach. The discovery was made by two doctors in Australia, Barry Marshall and Robin Warren, who were the first to isolate and identify the bacterium. It had long been assumed that the highly acidic environment of the stomach could not support any life form. But *H. pylori* lives in the protective mucous lining of the stomach, and it has evolved a special enzyme that allows it to generate ammonia as a means of neutralizing the stomach acid. It took more than a decade for the existence of *H. pylori* as a precipitating factor in stomach ulcers to be acknowledged. But it is now clear that the bacterium, by secreting toxic materials, helps to trigger damage to the stomach in a majority of the patients who develop ulcers. The bacterium is also common, however, in people who do not develop stomach ulcers – almost half of 40-year-old adults in Britain or the USA carry it. It appears to be the presence of *H. pylori*, along with other factors, such as stress or alcohol, that does the damage. Nowadays, gastric ulcers are routinely treated with H2 blockers or proton-pump inhibitors, along with an antibiotic to eradicate the *H. pylori* infection. Treatment with bismuth salts, or other drugs that help strengthen the mucous protective coating of the stomach, may also be given as part of a 'triple cocktail'.

Combating pain and inflammation

The immune system represents an immensely complex system of defence mechanisms that are called into play to counteract infections or injuries. The immune system is programmed to recognize any foreign materials and to activate the various defence mechanisms that are designed to destroy invading micro-organisms or to repair tissue damage. It does so by mobilizing antibodies – proteins that recognize foreign proteins or other large molecules and help to inactivate them. Binding of the foreign materials to antibodies helps to accelerate their disposal by the various classes of white blood cells, which attack, kill, and eventually engulf foreign cells or invading micro-organisms. White cells leave the bloodstream and concentrate in regions of tissue injury, where they help to remove dead and damaged cells and set up a local inflammatory response that is often painful. The immune system and white cells communicate with each other and with the rest of the body by means of a complex family of chemical signalling molecules known as chemokines and cytokines. These include a large family of proteins known as the interleukins and others with such exotic names as 'tumour necrosis factor' and 'interferons'. These molecules are generated when the immune system is activated and, among other things, they act on the brain to cause the so-called sickness syndrome, characterized by fever, sleepiness, and loss of appetite, symptoms that are well known to anyone who has suffered from a bout of flu or other infectious disease.

The immune system plays an essential role in combating enemies that would otherwise destroy us. Children born with defective immune systems are very vulnerable to infections and must be protected in restricted environments; and patients with AIDS eventually die because their immune system is disabled by the HIV virus. But this powerful defence system can also go wrong and turn against itself. A number of common human illnesses represent 'autoimmune' disorders, in which for some reason the immune system no longer recognizes some part of the body as 'self' and initiates an attack, with consequent inflammation and damage. Examples include arthritis, where joints become inflamed and painful and the cartilage and bone are gradually eroded; multiple sclerosis, a progressive disease of the nervous system in which the fatty material called myelin, which wraps around and insulates nerve fibres, is gradually attacked; and asthma, in which a chronic inflammation is set up in the lungs, leading to difficulties in breathing. Strangely, while people in the Western world are on the whole well fed and free of infectious diseases, the incidence of autoimmune disorders is going up, with particularly alarming increases in childhood asthma. One school of thought suggests that this is due to our living in a world that has become too clean and hygienic. Children are no longer exposed to dirt and germs as they used to be, and consequently the immune system has not got enough to do, and turns upon itself. Some have even advocated the deliberate exposure of children to a little dirt now and then – but this may be too extreme a remedy.

Fortunately there are many drugs available to treat the symptoms of pain and inflammation, although there are few that treat the underlying causes of these illnesses. The complex process of inflammation offers many targets for pharmacology. One of the oldest and most widely used of all drugs is aspirin. Aspirin is the drug name given to the chemical substance acetylsalicylic acid (Figure 11). It is a good example of how a relatively minor change in the parent chemical, salicylic acid, can lead to a dramatic improvement. The beneficial effects of extracts of willow bark (*Salix alba*) in reducing fevers have been known since the eighteenth century, and by the 1870s the effects of willow bark had been traced to the chemical salicylic acid. Methods for synthesizing salicylic acid were developed in Germany, and the Heyden Chemical Company initiated the commercial marketing of it as a medicine. It became widely used not only for fevers, but also for its effectiveness in reducing the pain associated with rheumatism, arthritis, headaches, and neuralgias. Salicyclic acid, however, was far from the ideal medicine – it was administered as a solution with a vile and bitter

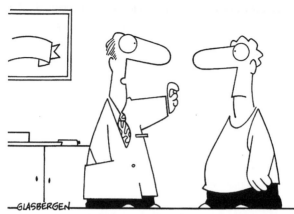

"To prevent a heart attack, take one aspirin every day.
Take it out for a jog, then take it to the gym,
then take it for a bike ride...."

10.

taste, which often caused the patient to vomit, and it caused severe irritation to the lining of the stomach that could lead to life-threatening bleeding ulcers. It was the chemist Felix Hoffmann and the pharmacologist Heinrich Dreser, working in the Bayer Company in Germany, who solved these problems by synthesizing the acetyl derivative of salicylic acid, aspirin, in 1898. In a scientific paper published in 1899 Dreser showed that in animals aspirin retained the excellent pain-relieving and fever-reducing properties of the parent substance and at the same time offered a safer and more convenient medicine. Aspirin lacks the bitter taste of the parent salicyclic acid, but does not dissolve readily in water, and so the Bayer Company decided to supply the compound in the form of compressed tablets, which would disintegrate into powder form in the stomach. Aspirin thus became the first major medicine to be sold in tablet form. Launched at the turn of the twentieth century, it became the 'drug of the century'. It was widely used to treat many sorts of pain, and the availability of a safe and non-addictive painkiller was very welcome at a time when morphine was the only alternative available. For a while the Bayer Company enjoyed a monopoly position and reaped huge commercial profits from the drug, but after 1918 many other companies were able to manufacture and market the drug, as the original patents expired. This led to intensely competitive marketing campaigns, the so-called aspirin wars, to sell what became one of the most widely used of all medicines.

New medical uses continue to be discovered for aspirin. One of its many effects is to act on specialized cells in the blood known as platelets, which are important in blood clotting. By disabling the platelet-clotting mechanism, aspirin makes blood less likely to clot – and, since unwanted blood clots can initiate heart attacks or a stroke, taking a low dose of aspirin every day is recommended to patients who are at risk of these events. The mechanism underlying the actions of aspirin remained unknown until the British pharmacologist John (now Sir John) Vane and his colleagues showed that it acts as an inhibitor of a key enzyme in the inflammatory mechanism called cyclo-oxygenase. This enzyme generates an inflammatory mediator known as prostaglandin, which triggers pain and other aspects of inflammation. By inhibiting the formation of prostaglandin, aspirin reduces pain and dampens down the overall inflammatory process. Vane showed that not only aspirin but

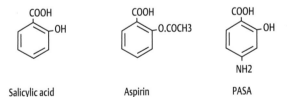

Salicylic acid   Aspirin   PASA

11. Chemical structures of drug molecules. Small alterations in chemical structure can produce major changes in drug activity. The addition of an acetic acid group to the natural product salicylic acid led to aspirin, a far less toxic compound that was much easier to administer in tablet form. Fifty years later in another laboratory the addition of an amino (NH2) group produced para-amino-salicylic acid (PASA) one of the first effective drugs for treating tuberculosis.

all the other so-called non-steroidal anti-inflammatory drugs (NSAIDs) that had been developed since aspirin (for example, ibuprofen, ketoflac, and indomethacin) also worked by the same mechanism. Vane was awarded the Nobel Prize for Physiology and Medicine in 1982 in recognition of this seminal discovery.

The aspirin story continues to develop. A new class of NSAIDs was introduced at the end of the twentieth century that is as effective as the previous drugs as pain-relievers and anti-inflammatory agents, but that is much less prone to cause gastric irritation and bleeding. These remain the most common and serious of the unwanted side effects associated with aspirin and the other aspirin-like drugs. Although these side effects are rarely serious, they can become so, and, because so many millions of people take aspirin and other NSAIDS, several thousand people die each year as a result of severe drug-induced gastric bleeding. The new drugs target a newly discovered form of the cyclo-oxygenase enzyme, known as COX-2. Unlike the previously studied enzyme, now known as COX-1, the COX-2 enzyme is generated only in response to inflammation or injury. It is thus an ideal target for anti-inflammatory drugs. Unlike the older NSAIDS, which inhibit both enzymes equally, the new drugs selectively inhibit only the COX-2 enzyme. The COX-2 enzyme is not present in the cells lining the stomach where COX-1 is found, so the COX-2 inhibitors do not cause gastric irritation and bleeding. The COX-2 inhibitors look set to be the blockbusters for the twenty-first century that aspirin was 100 years earlier. They offer the possibility of safer pain relief for millions of elderly patients, for whom the earlier generation of NSAIDS can prove dangerous. Sales of the two COX-2 blockers already launched, Vioxx® and Celebrex®, already exceeded $3 billion in 2000.

Other aspirin-like drugs exist, the most widely used of which is paracetamol (marketed as Panadol or Tylenol). Paracetamol is an effective painkiller and reduces fevers, but is safer than aspirin. It does not cause gastric irritation and can be given to children or elderly patients. The mechanism of action is somewhat obscure, but it is thought to act by inhibiting the cyclo-oxygenase enzyme in the brain rather than in peripheral tissues. There is a danger, however, as in an overdose paracetamol can cause serious damage to the liver and kidneys. Because it is so widely used, there are paracetamol-related deaths every year – sometimes as a result of deliberate suicidal overdosing.

For more severe forms of pain, often associated with such terminal illnesses as cancer, morphine or morphine-like drugs, the 'opiates', remain the most effective options. Morphine acts on specific opiate receptor sites in the brain and spinal cord to dampen the flow of nerve impulses in nerve tracts that carry 'pain' information into the brain. These receptors are not there to recognize the plant-derived drug, but they are part of the body's own pain defence system. The opiate receptors are normally activated by naturally occurring chemicals known as endorphins (*endo*genous m*orphines*). These chemicals are released particularly in conditions of stress or emergency when fight or flight is more important than feeling pain. Thus, the footballer injured on the field or the soldier wounded in battle does not feel the pain immediately. There are now many synthetic chemical drugs that act on the same receptors as morphine, and some of these are many times more potent than morphine itself (for example, fentanyl). Morphine itself, however, continues to be widely used, and new slow-release preparations make it possible to control most forms of pain with a drug regime that administers a dose once or twice a day. There are problems associated with the repeated use of morphine and related opiates, however. Doctors are often frightened of using these drugs except in the terminally ill in case they create drug addiction (see Chapter 4), although this rarely if ever happens. A more practical problem is that the repeated use of morphine-like drugs leads to the development of tolerance, so that higher and higher drug doses are needed, and eventually the patient may no longer obtain adequate pain relief. There remains a real need for better medicines to control severe chronic pain.

Healing the damaged mind

One of the most remarkable advances in pharmacology in the latter half of the twentieth century was the discovery and widespread use of drugs that help to treat the symptoms of mental disorders.

The availability of drugs that ameliorate the symptoms of schizophrenia, depression, and anxiety has had a major impact on the way in which we view these diseases: they are seen increasingly as having an organic basis. The drugs have also led to radical changes in the management of mental illnesses – leading, for example, to the closure of the mental hospitals as places where dangerous mad people had be kept locked away from the rest of society.

Virtually all of the drugs used in psychiatry act in one way or another on the chemical messenger systems in the brain. The billions of nerve cells in the brain communicate with each other in complex neural circuits. Nerve cells maintain a small electrical potential between the inside of the cell and the outside world, and the discharge of this 'battery' allows them to transmit electrical impulses along their elongated fibres. When the electrical pulse reaches the vicinity of the next cell in the circuit, however, transmission from cell to cell is no longer electrical but chemical. The nerve impulse arriving at a nerve fibre ending causes the discharge of a minute amount of one or other of the many different chemical messenger substances used in the brain. The chemical acts on receptor proteins on the surface of the target cell to cause either an excitation or an inhibition of the activity of that cell (it is as important to have OFF signals as it is to have ON signals) (Figure 12).

More than fifty different chemicals are used in this way as messenger molecules, and each is recognized by its own specific cell surface receptors. This offers many different targets for drug intervention, either to boost the function of a particular chemical messenger or to

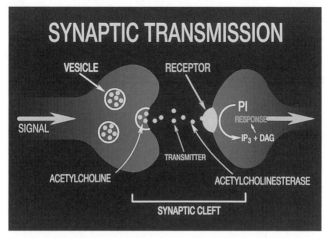

12. Chemical transmission in the nervous system. Nerve cells (neurons) transmit minute electrical impulses down their cable-like fibres (axons). When the impulses reach the ending of the fibre they trigger the release of bursts of a neurotransmitter chemical which activate the target cell. Many drugs that act on the nervous system do so by either mimicking neurotransmitter molecules or by blocking their actions on target.

block its actions. The first effective drugs used to treat clinical depression were compounds that act by enhancing the activity of chemicals known as monoamines in the brain. The two chemicals that appear particularly relevant for depression are noradrenaline (norepinephrine) and serotonin. Each of these plays a role in modulating the activity of the thinking part of the brain, the cerebral cortex. Noradrenaline helps to alert the brain to interesting events going on in the outside world, and serotonin plays a key role in determining the emotional state and mood.

The first safe and effective antidepressant drugs were discovered in the 1950s: imipramine in Europe by the Swiss company CIBA-GEIGY, and amitriptyline by the American company Merck. These drugs boost monoamine function in the brain. After release from nerve endings,

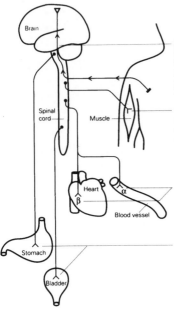

Sensory nerves carry information to the brain from the skin about touch, temperature, pressure, and pain, and from the joints and muscles about the position of our body and limbs

'Voluntary' muscles in the body and limbs have nerves which release the transmitter acetylcholine. It acts on nicotinic or 'N' receptors

Most organs have 'sympathetic' nerves which release the transmitter norepinephrine. This can act on α or β receptors

A third group of nerves, the 'parasympathetic' nerves, release acetylcholine as their transmitter but this now acts on muscarinic or 'M' receptors to control involuntary muscles such as those in the heart and bladder

13. Peripheral nervous system. In addition to sensory nerves and those contracting the voluntary muscles, we have two types of involuntary (autonomic) nerves: the 'sympathetic' and the 'parasympathetic'.

noradrenaline and serotonin are inactivated by an unusual recapture mechanism whereby they are pumped back into the nerve endings from which they had been released by means of a specific transporter protein located in the cell membrane of the nerve. The antidepressants imipramine and amitriptyline act by inhibiting these amine pump mechanisms, thus prolonging the actions of released monoamines. Dr Julius Axelrod, working at the US National Institute of Mental Health, was the first to discover the monoamine uptake mechanisms, and the actions of the antidepressants on them – for which he was awarded the Nobel Prize for Physiology and Medicine in 1970. Imipramine and amitriptyline proved hugely popular and continue to be widely used. During the 1980s and 1990s, however, even more successful antidepressants were discovered. These target more selectively just the monoamine transporter for serotonin, leaving other monoamine transporters untouched. The serotonin-selective reuptake inhibitors (SSRIs), epitomized by Prozac® (fluoxetine), are even safer to use than the older drugs, which could prove dangerous in an overdose. Prozac and related SSRIs have captured an ever-increasing market for antidepressant medicines – valued at more than $11 billion in 1999. Two SSRIs are currently among the top ten best selling of all pharmaceutical products. The availability of safe and effective drugs has demonstrated that clinical depression affects far larger numbers of people than was hitherto thought.

Anxiety often accompanies depression, and it occurs in many different forms. At one extreme are patients who suffer from severe anxiety and panic attacks. They may experience several frightening panic attacks every week, often prompted by some particular phobia – fear of open spaces, or entering the supermarket, or social occasions. There are many milder forms of phobia and anxiety – often associated with generalized anxiety and insomnia. The most effective anti-anxiety drugs (tranquillizers) are the benzodiazepines, epitomized by diazepam (Valium®). The benzodiazepines have a remarkable calming effect on anxious people, and they help to restore normal sleep patterns. Valium®

was the best-selling drug in the pharmaceutical world for more than a decade in the 1960s and 1970s, and earned a fortune for the parent Swiss company, Hoffmann la Roche. It was followed by many imitators, all sharing the same pharmacological mechanism, which is to enhance the actions of the key inhibitory brain chemical messenger GABA. Benzodiazepines are also widely used to combat insomnia, and for this purpose very short-acting drugs have been designed – so that they do not leave the patient with a sedated 'hangover' effect on waking next morning. Like most psychopharmaceuticals, however, there is a downside to the repeated use of benzodiazepines. Some patients can become addicted to the drugs, so that they find it difficult to stop taking them. If drug treatment is stopped, it can lead to a period of rebound associated with increased anxiety and sleep disturbance. On the whole, though, the benzodiazepines represent a remarkably safe group of drugs that have benefited many millions of patients.

We all occasionally suffer from bouts of anxiety or depression, so we feel some empathy for the patients who suffer from the extreme forms of these conditions. The madness of schizophrenia is much more difficult for us to understand. Schizophrenia affects about 1 per cent of the population. It develops after puberty in early adult life, and is often a lifelong illness. The symptoms are varied and bizarre; no two patients will be quite the same. Key symptoms include: auditory hallucinations – often hearing voices talking about the patient in the third person; irrational delusions; feelings of persecution and paranoia; inability to express appropriate emotions; incoherent thought processes and language; withdrawal from social contacts and immobility. The illness often leaves the sufferer incapable of normal work or other daily activities, and the delusions may lead the patient to irrational and dangerous acts of violence towards others. The discovery of drugs that tackle some of these key symptoms has been a big advance in the treatment of schizophrenia. The first breakthrough was an accidental discovery. In the early 1950s two French physicians, J. Delay and P. Deniker, noted the remarkable calming effects of a new drug, chlorpromazine, which was initially tested as an agent to be given to patients prior to major surgery to relax them. They tested the drug in patients suffering from mania and found it to be remarkably effective, and this led to tests in schizophrenic patients, where again chlorpromazine had remarkable effects in calming agitated patients, without putting them to sleep – it was a tranquillizer, not a crude sedative. Chlorpromazine rapidly came into widespread use on both sides of the Atlantic as a new and effective treatment for schizophrenia. Many other effective anti-schizophrenia agents followed chlorpromazine, including the very potent drug haloperidol, discovered by the gifted drug-discoverer Paul Janssen in Belgium. Some of these drugs were up to a thousand times more potent than chlorpromazine, so that it proved possible to deliver enough drug to last for several weeks in one single dose – usually given by means of an injection of the drug in an oily fluid into a muscle. This 'depot injection' remains in the muscle and slowly releases an active drug. In this way it has proved possible to treat schizophrenia in outpatient clinics, in which the drug is administered once or twice a month. The availability of such treatments has been one of the factors that has led to the gradual disappearance of the Victorian mental hospitals, in which patients with schizophrenia were formerly locked away.

Discovering how anti-schizophrenic drugs act in the brain has been one of the achievements of the new subject of 'psychopharmacology', and two of the pioneers in this field, Arvid Carlsson in Sweden and Paul Greengard in the USA, were awarded the Nobel Prize for Physiology and Medicine in 2000. They helped to show that the key target for all of the effective drugs in this class is one of the monoamine chemical messengers called dopamine. This chemical is also associated with another brain disorder, Parkinson's disease, in which the nerve cells that make and release dopamine gradually degenerate, leaving the sufferer unable to initiate movements, and with rigid limbs often accompanied by a tremor. Giving the drug L-DOPA, which enters the brain, treats Parkinson's disease; L-DOPA is converted to dopamine to replace the missing brain chemical. The drugs used to treat schizophrenia, however, act in the opposite way to block the actions of dopamine at its receptors in the brain. It is thus no surprise to learn that one of the adverse side effects of these drugs is to cause symptoms similar to those seen in Parkinson's disease, or conversely that an overdose of L-DOPA can cause psychotic symptoms. The problem of side effects similar to Parkinson's disease has been largely overcome, however, in a new generation of anti-schizophrenic drugs, which remain as effective as the older drugs in combating the psychotic symptoms of the illness but are less prone to cause unwanted Parkinsonian side effects. The newer drugs combine blockade of dopamine receptors with another pharmacological action, blocking one of the receptors used by the monoamine serotonin. By this dual blockade the drugs avoid the Parkinsonian side effects. Schizophrenia is a fairly common illness, and drug treatment, although not a cure, has been of great benefit to millions of patients worldwide.

Much remains to be learned about how drugs act on the brain to produce such dramatic effects on such complex conditions as depression, anxiety, or psychosis. In nearly all cases, for example, the beneficial effects of the drugs are seen only after they have been administered for some weeks – whereas the actual pharmacological action (that is, the blockade of serotonin uptake, the antagonism of dopamine receptors, and so on) is immediate. It seems that the immediate action of the drug triggers some longer-term processes that lead to a gradual correction of mental imbalance – by mechanisms still unknown.

There is also great interest in discovering new and better classes of drugs to treat mental disorders, and in particular to treat the growing problem of Alzheimer's disease and other forms of senile dementia. So far there has been little progress in the treatment of such disorders (see Chapter 6).

Plagues and pestilences: combating the unseen invaders

Throughout human history infectious diseases have plagued us. As the human species became more and more numerous and lived in increasingly high densities in towns and cities, we became a fertile breeding ground for the many species of bacteria, fungi, and viruses that have evolved specifically to take advantage of *Homo sapiens*. For most of human history we have had no effective medical means of combating the ravages of infectious diseases, and had to rely instead on the sophisticated defences of our own immune system. When the immune system is overwhelmed, however, often in response to exposure to an unfamiliar infection that has spread from some other part of the world, the consequences can be lethal. The spread of bubonic plague (the 'Black Death') throughout Europe in the Middle Ages, for example, led to the death of as many as half of the population in many countries. Even in the twentieth century, the 'Spanish flu' epidemic killed some thirty million people within six months in 1918 – twice as many as had died in the First World War.

It was not until the seventeenth century that Robert Hooke in London first looked at a drop of water under the newly discovered microscope and was astonished to find it seething with millions of tiny living organisms, quite invisible to the naked eye. But it took another 200 years for the link to be made between such micro-organisms and human disease. The first evidence that disease could be spread from person to person came only in the nineteenth century. At first the only means of applying this new knowledge was to improve standards of hygiene; this was particularly important in hospitals, where doctors spread diseases from patient to patient – often because they did not wash their hands between treating patients. Improved antiseptic conditions in operating theatres also helped – as did the construction of systems of mains sewerage in towns and cities. Until the late nineteenth century it was certainly not safe to drink the water from the pump or tap in Britain. The only drinks that were safe were beer or tea – because in both cases the water had been boiled before it was used to prepare the drink.

Although some of the ancient herbal medicines contained active drugs that helped to combat certain infectious conditions, there was little available in the medicine cabinet until the twentieth century. Reference has already been made to the pioneering work of Paul Ehrlich, who discovered arsphenamine, the first effective treatment for the bacterium causing syphilis. This was followed in the 1930s by the discovery of the sulphonamides as a new and powerful class of antibacterial agents. Then followed the era of antibiotics – with the often-told story of Alexander Fleming finding in 1928 that a mould had killed bacteria on an experimental bacterial growth plate left by the window of his laboratory in London. It took another ten years for Howard Florey, Norman Heatley, and Ernst Chain in Oxford to identify the antibacterial substance as penicillin, and to treat the first patient in 1941. Fleming, Florey, and Chain shared the Nobel Prize for Physiology and Medicine in 1945 for their discovery of penicillin. Penicillin proved to be of major importance in the Second World War in treating infected battle wounds, and production was taken over from war-stricken Britain to America, where the drug was made on a large scale for the first time by Merck and other pharmaceutical companies. Penicillin was to be followed by many other powerful antibiotic drugs, which have revolutionized our ability to combat such killer diseases as pneumonia, tuberculosis, and cholera. The antibiotics were followed in turn later in the twentieth century by the first effective drugs for treating virus diseases. How do these miracle drugs work?

Antibacterial and anti-fungal drugs

The ideal drug for treating an infectious disease is one that targets some aspect of biology that is unique to the bacterium or fungus, so that the invading organism can be killed without damaging the human host. The most effective anti-microbial drugs do just that. Bacteria are tiny particles of living matter; they are protected from the outside world by a fairly tough cell membrane – without which they are very vulnerable and cannot survive and multiply. Many antibiotics work by disrupting the ability of the bacteria to synthesize and put together the various sugar and protein components that make up the cell wall. This disables the bacteria, as they cannot reproduce and the immune system can then clear any remaining infection. Penicillin works in this manner and so do the more than twenty different synthetic analogues of penicillin now available. Another important group of antibiotics, the cephalosporins, a class that includes more than twenty-five different drugs, are chemically distinct from the penicillins but act in the same way as cell wall inhibitors, as do vancomycin and bacitracin.

Other classes of antibacterial agents make use of other differences between bacteria and their hosts. The sulphonamides, for example, interfere with the synthesis of folic acid by bacteria. Folic acid is an essential vitamin that acts as a catalyst for various chemical reactions in all living cells, but, whereas we get the vitamin in our diet, the bacterium must synthesize it. Interfering with this process makes it impossible for the bacteria to grow. Although the sulphonamides were discovered a long time ago, there have been many improvements and some sixteen drugs in this class are still available and widely used. Tetracyclines and the related aminoglycoside antibiotics interfere with another vital life process – the synthesis of proteins. They target the protein synthesis machinery of bacteria, which is different from that of mammals so the drugs do no harm to the host. This class of drugs also includes streptomycin, the first effective antibiotic for the treatment of tuberculosis (see Chapter 6). The macrolide antibiotics also employ this mechanism of action; this class includes erythromycin, one of the most effective drugs for treating pneumonia. Yet other drugs target the synthesis of nucleic acids by bacteria – another essential feature of life; these include the quinolones and rifampicin.

Infections can be caused by various species of fungi as well as by bacteria. These affect particularly those areas of the body with surfaces exposed to the outside world: skin, lungs, throat, vagina, urinary tract, and so on. Drugs that act against fungal infections, like the antibacterial drugs, target features that are unique to the biology of the invading fungi. As with bacteria, fungi synthesize a tough cell wall and a number of anti-fungal agents interfere with the synthesis or function of this – making use particularly of a cholesterol-like molecule ergosterol, which is a unique component of fungal cell walls, as a target. Amphotericin, nystatin, and imidazoles act in this way. Other anti-fungal drugs target features of nucleic acid or protein synthesis unique to fungi.

Drugs to treat virus infections

Taking antibiotics will not cure the common cold, nor will they alleviate the symptoms of flu or influence the course of AIDS infections. These and many other infectious diseases are caused not by bacteria but by viruses. Viruses are the smallest and most simplified forms of life.

Viruses have dispensed with much of the biochemical machinery that other organisms need to live and to reproduce; they do not need this machinery, because they live as parasites within the living cells of their host. Most viruses simply consist of a length of nucleic acid – which carries encoded information about how to make more virus particles – wrapped up in a protein coat. Virus particles infect cells by attaching themselves to the surface of the cell and gaining entry. Once inside the host cell, they shed their protein coat and hijack the biochemistry of the host cell, diverting it to the synthesis of new virus nucleic acid and protein molecules, which will eventually be assembled into millions of new virus particles. The host cell is then killed and the new virus particles released for another round of infection.

Designing effective anti-viral drugs is difficult, as the virus has so few unique features. It uses the normal biochemical machinery of the host, so targeting this is likely to cause damage to the host. The first effective anti-viral drugs were discovered only in the latter part of the twentieth century. Some target the enzyme DNA polymerase, which is needed for the replication of the nucleic acid DNA; without this the virus cannot replicate. But this enzyme is present in all cells of the host. The clever trick here was to design drugs that are not themselves active inhibitors of the DNA polymerase enzyme, but which are selectively converted to such inhibitors only in the virus-infected cells of the host – which contain a viral enzyme that converts the drug. This concept of using an inert drug that is converted in the body to an active agent is an example of the so-called pro-drug strategy. This produced the anti-viral agent acyclovir and a dozen or so later derivatives of it, discoveries that earned the American scientists Gertrude Elion and George Hitchings the Nobel Prize for Physiology and Medicine in 1988. Another important anti-viral drug is zidovudine (AZT); this also impairs the replication of viral nucleic acids, fooling the viral enzyme into incorporating AZT into its own nucleic acid, which can then no longer replicate.

The virus responsible for AIDS, the human immunodeficiency virus (HIV), is one of the most spectacular success stories in viral evolution. This virus has adapted to live in the most numerous large animal on earth (*Homo sapiens*) and it selectively attacks the very cells in the immune system of its host – the T-cells – that are normally in the front line in the body's fight against infections. Furthermore, HIV is spread mainly by sexual contact – one of the most popular forms of human behaviour. The virus gradually destroys the ability of the immune system to mount any further attack, and the body succumbs to the virus and to a variety of other infections – which can include viruses that cause cancers. The first modest success in treating HIV infections came from the use of the anti-viral drugs that target viral nucleic acid replication, but the most successful drugs have emerged in recent years with a different mechanism. They target an enzyme that is unique to the HIV virus. When the virus replicates, the information encoded in the viral nucleic acid is read out as a single long protein, which has to be cut into several different functional protein units. This cutting is done by a special viral enzyme known as HIV protease, and a family of protease inhibitors now represent the most effective drugs in the battle against AIDS. A problem in the treatment of this and other viral diseases is that the virus can mutate to a form that is resistant to the drug. This is evolution running at high speed. During a prolonged period of HIV infection, more than a thousand million particles of HIV virus are generated every day and most are killed by the immune system. The opportunities for a small number of mutant virus particles to arise by chance are thus very high, and if some of these mutants have an advantage, for example, in being resistant to ongoing anti-viral drug treatment, they will survive and multiply. To combat this problem of drug resistance, it is now common to use a protease inhibitor as part of a cocktail of drugs, together with one or more of the earlier anti-viral agents (for example, AZT) to make it more difficult for drug resistance to emerge. So far this strategy seems to be working. In the rich countries of the world the life expectancy of people who are HIV-positive has improved dramatically. They or their insurance companies can afford the $10,000 a year or so that it costs to use one of the 'triple-therapy' cocktails of anti-HIV drugs now available. Between 1996 when the protease inhibitors were introduced and 1998, deaths attributable to AIDS in the USA dropped by more than 70 per cent and AIDS no longer ranks among the top ten causes of death. It is too early to claim a final victory, however. The spread of the HIV virus in the body may be largely controlled by the new treatments, but pockets of infection can remain for long periods – for example, in the brain, where the virus is protected by the blood–brain barrier. The 'triple-therapy' drug treatment regime may need to be continued indefinitely, and carries its own risks of toxicity. It is also likely that mutant strains of HIV will continue to emerge that are resistant to even the most powerful drugs currently available, and this means that there will be a continuing need to discover and develop new anti-viral drugs. People living in the poorer parts of the world cannot afford treatment with even a single anti-AIDS drug, let alone the expensive triple cocktails used in the West.

By the end of the twentieth century more than twenty million people in Africa alone were infected with HIV, and their prospects are very bleak.

Killing parasites

As with bacteria, fungi, and viruses, a wide range of parasitic animals have found *Homo sapiens* to be an attractive host in which to live. These range from single-celled organisms, known as Protozoa, to larger parasitic creatures (flatworms, roundworms, hookworms tapeworms, and so on). Infections are commonest in tropical and subtropical regions, where they can have devastating consequences. The protozoan Trypanosomes, for example, infect cattle in West Africa, making large areas of land unsuitable for cattle farming. In humans, other strains of Trypanosomes invade the brain and cause damage that leads to 'sleeping sickness'. In other tropical countries in Africa, Toxocara or Onchocerca parasitic worms infect the eye and lead to 'river blindness'. A powerful new drug, ivermectin, first discovered as a treatment for the parasites that commonly infect horses and farm animals, can combat the latter condition. Ivermectin has been made available to the World Health Organisation for a campaign to fight river blindness in Africa. A single tablet of this wonder drug taken at six-month intervals can protect children and adults against the terrible consequences of infection with this parasite. In general, though, the pharmaceutical armoury available to treat parasitic infection is not particularly strong. These are diseases that affect mainly the poorer parts of the world, and there is little economic motivation for pharmaceutical companies to invest heavily in research on tropical diseases. The most important example of such neglect is the case of malaria, the commonest and most deadly of all parasitic diseases. Malaria is caused by a group of protozoan parasites known as Plasmodium. Infection is passed from person to person through the bite of an Anopheles mosquito and the parasite grows initially in the liver and then in red blood cells, from which it is eventually released, causing a sudden bout of fever and disability. As many as 400 million people are infected with malaria every year and some two million of them die from the disease. More than 10,000 cases occur every year in Western tourists visiting malaria-infected regions. Fortunately there are some effective drugs to treat malaria. The oldest of these is quinine, first discovered in the bark of the Cinchona tree in the seventeenth century and later isolated and purified in the nineteenth century in Paris. Quinine and its derivatives chloroquine and mefloquine kill the malarial parasites in red blood cells by a complex mechanism that involves a chemical reaction with the red blood pigment haemoglobin. A few other drugs are available: pyrimethamine and proguanil inhibit folic acid synthesis in the parasite – a mechanism similar to that of the sulphonamides in bacteria – and primaquine attacks the parasite in its early stage of development in the liver. Unfortunately, however, drug resistance has become an increasing problem in combating malaria, and in some parts of the world the parasite has already evolved resistance to such an extent that few effective drugs remain available. There is an urgent need to discover new drug treatments for this killer disease.

Resistance to antibiotics

This enquiry has been an alarming experience, which leaves us convinced that resistance to antibiotics and other anti-infective agents constitutes a major threat to public health, and ought to be recognised as such more widely than it is at present.

(UK House of Lords – 1997)

One of the biggest problems in the drug treatment of disease lies in the very area in which there has been such spectacular success in the past century – the use of antibiotics and other drugs to treat infectious diseases. The widespread use of these drugs has led inevitably to the evolution of new strains of bacteria, viruses, and parasites that are drug resistant. That such evolution could occur so rapidly may at first sight seem surprising. However, infectious organisms such as bacteria and viruses grow and reproduce very rapidly in the human body; bacterial numbers can double within a few minutes. During the course of an infection that can last weeks or months, thousands of generations of bacteria will be generated, most of which will be killed by antibacterial drugs or by the immune system. But a tiny proportion of mutant cells that are drug resistant will have an enormous advantage over the others, and they are likely to survive and prosper. Because it is so tempting for doctors to prescribe antibiotics to every patient who turns up with some mild infection and fever, there is a great deal of unnecessary prescribing. In hospitals antibiotics are again almost universally used for sick patients and hospitals have proved to be hotbeds for the evolution and breeding of antibiotic-resistant strains of micro-organism. To quote an example from the House of Lords report:

> Staphylococci are omnipresent on our skins; they are normally benign but capable of causing infections ranging from a boil to life-threatening septicaemia. Methicillin-resistant *Staphylococcus aureus* (MRSA), often also resistant to many other antibiotics, has become highly prevalent in many hospitals and nursing homes. Only vancomycin and related drugs, toxic, expensive and not always effective agents, remain for their treatment; and the first isolates of vancomycin-resistant *S. aureus* (VRSA) have already been reported in Japan and the USA.

To make matters worse, modern farming methods, in which animals are kept at high densities in confined spaces, are dependent on the widespread use of antibiotics to prevent otherwise inevitable infections. In many cases farm animals are treated indiscriminately with antibiotics to protect them against infections and thus to increase their growth rates.

The molecular devices that micro-organisms have evolved to combat antibiotics are truly remarkable. Following the introduction of penicillin, some mutant strains of bacteria started to make a new enzyme 'penicillinase' that was capable of degrading and inactivating the drug.

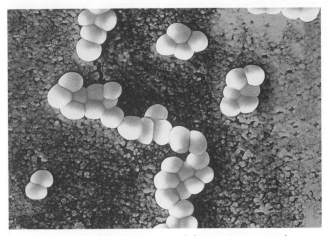

14. Individual cells of the bacterium *Staphylococcus aureus*, greatly enlarged. This bacterium can cause serious infections in wounds or in the lung, leading to pneumonia. Strains of this bacterium that are resistant to many antibiotics are common in modern hospitals.

The response of the drug industry to these penicillin-resistant strains was to develop synthetic derivatives of penicillin that were resistant to attack by penicillinase. This strategy was defeated in turn, as new strains of bacteria evolved with a form of the enzyme that could attack the newer drugs – and so the game of cat and mouse goes on. Other devices that confer drug resistance include the modification of the prime target of the drug to make it no longer effective. Thus, for example, strains of bacteria have evolved that use an entirely new way of synthesizing their cell wall materials – thus making them resistant to the many different antibiotics that work by blocking cell wall synthesis. An even more remarkable evolution has been the development of a gene called 'Multiple Drug Resistance' (MDR), which consists of a molecular pump mechanism that can actively expel a number of different antibiotics from the bacterial cell – thus conferring resistance to a whole group of antibiotics. Bacteria have also proved more adept than previously thought in transferring these antibiotic resistance genes

Examples of valuable antibiotic therapies now lost or imperilled by the spread of resistance

Organism, disease	Agents lost or threatened
Pneumococcus pneumonia, otitis, meningitis	Penicillin, many others
Meningococcus meningitis, septicaemia	Sulphonamides (penicillin)
Haemophilus influenzae, meningitis	Ampicillin, chloramphenicol
Staphylococcus aureus, wound infection, sepsis	Penicillin, penicillinase-resistant penicillins
Salmonella typhi, typhoid fever	Most relevant agents
Shigella spp., bacillary dysentery	Most relevant agents
Gonococcus, gonorrhoea	Sulphonamides, penicillin, tetracycline (ciprofloxacin)
Plasmodium falciparum, severe malaria	Chloroquine, pyrimethamine (mefloquine quinine)
E. coli (coliforms), urinary infection, septicaemia	Ampicillin, trimethoprim, others

UK House of Lords, Select Committee on Science and Technology, Report on 'Resistance to Antibiotics' (UK House of Lords, 1997) from one species of bacteria to another. The evolutionary pressures on the development and spread of these genes has been intense, and so far bacteria have scored some ominous successes – making some infectious diseases increasingly difficult to treat. The probability that an inpatient stay in a hospital will lead to an infection with an antibiotic-resistant bacterium is increasing alarmingly every year. The battle against infectious disease will go on indefinitely. Not only are drug-resistant strains of micro-organism constantly evolving; we are faced with a stream of hitherto little-known infectious diseases, spread to the Western world by the increasing global mobility of *Homo sapiens.*

From having almost no effective drugs to treat infectious disease at the start of the twentieth century, by 2000 several hundred were available. Particular drugs have been found to be the best for individual infectious diseases, and they have become widely used – some say far too widely used in modern medicine. This group of drugs, perhaps more than any other, has affected the health of people who are fortunate enough to live in the developed world, and they have largely taken away ancient fears of these infectious diseases. In the poorer regions of the globe, however, infectious diseases are still important killers. Some twenty million people die in such countries every year from these diseases; five million from respiratory infections, three million from tuberculosis, and three million from cholera and other diarrhoeal diseases.

The examples illustrated above hopefully give some impression of the important role that new twentieth-century drugs have played in changing the way that medicine is practised. There have been many other advances in the drug treatment of human illness, and the impact that some of these have had on all of our lives will be reviewed again in Chapter 6.

Chapter 4
Recreational drugs

The total annual worldwide market for all medical drugs is approximately $250 billion, but the market for recreational drugs is probably at least ten times greater. People in both rich and poor countries seem to have a constant desire to alter their state of consciousness. They use stimulant drugs that allow them to stay awake and dance the night away, sedatives to calm their anxieties, and intoxicants to experience new forms of consciousness and to forget the troubles of everyday life.

The problem is that recreational drug use can lead to abuse. One of the insidious aspects of recreational drug use is that it can all too easily lead to the user becoming dependent on the drug. In modern usage the term 'dependence' is often used rather than 'addiction'. The symptoms of dependence may include 'tolerance' (the need to take larger and larger doses of the substance to achieve the desired effect), and 'physical dependence' (an altered physical state induced by the substance that produces physical 'withdrawal symptoms', such as nausea, vomiting, seizures, and headache, when substance use is terminated); but neither of these is necessary or sufficient for the diagnosis of substance dependence. Dependence can be defined in some instances entirely in terms of 'psychological dependence'; this differs from earlier thinking on these concepts, which tended to equate addiction with physical dependence.

The dependent drug-user may continue to take excessive amounts of the drug, even though it is clearly damaging to work, health, and family. Fortunately, not everyone who takes a recreational drug becomes dependent on it. It is possible that there are people with an 'addictive personality' who are more susceptible than others. Drugs differ in their dependence liability – ranging from high risk in the case of cocaine, heroin, and nicotine to lower risk in the case of alcohol, cannabis, and amphetamines. What changes go on in the brain during the development of drug dependence remain a mystery. The process requires the repeated use of drugs over prolonged periods, so scientists think of it as involving a change in the pattern of genes that are switched on (or off) in the brain, but just what the critical changes are is not yet clear. Animals can become dependent on recreational drugs, and research on animal brains has suggested that there may be some common mechanisms that are triggered by a number of different drugs. Although the primary sites of action of heroin, amphetamines, nicotine, cocaine, and cannabis in the brain are all different, these drugs share an ability to promote the release of the chemical messenger dopamine in certain brain regions. Although this is not necessarily akin to triggering a 'pleasure' mechanism, it is thought that the drug-induced release of dopamine may be an important signal that prompts the animal or person to seek continued drug use.

Alcohol, nicotine, and caffeine: the three big legal drugs

Alcohol

Alcohol is the oldest of all recreational drugs, and it is widely consumed in the Western world. The production of wines, beers, and distilled spirits is a very large industry, with worldwide sales of more than $300 billion. In most Western countries more than 80 per cent of the adult population will admit to having tried alcohol, and about 50 per cent are regular users. The consumption of alcohol continues to increase, and the range of alcoholic drinks is constantly widening – with, for example, sweet 'alcopop' drinks to attract the younger consumer – and in many countries alcoholic products are available twenty-four hours a day in supermarkets. The alcohol industry spends large amounts of money on advertising to encourage the sales of its products. The consumption of alcoholic drinks is deeply embedded in the culture of many countries: the special atmosphere of the traditional English pub or the German beer garden; the custom of drinking wine with the meal in France and Italy; the ice-cold aquavit of the Scandinavian cold table; and the universal champagne at the wedding reception.

Exactly how alcohol acts in the brain to produce initially a state of excitement and intoxication and later sedation is not precisely understood. Scientists believe that the key actions of alcohol target the two principal chemical messenger systems in the neural circuits of the brain. Alcohol enhances the actions of the main OFF signal, GABA, and partially blocks the main ON signal, L-glutamate. But there is more to it than that: the pleasurable intoxicant actions of alcohol seem to be due in part to its ability to stimulate opiate mechanisms in the brain – the same ones that are stimulated more directly and more aggressively by heroin. The drug naltrexone acts as an antagonist of the opiate receptors in the brain. It has been used successfully in treating heroin addicts, and more recently it has been shown to be effective in treating alcoholics. The drug removes the pleasurable effects of both heroin and alcohol, making it easier for the dependent user to quit.

The majority of drinkers are able to indulge in alcohol without damaging themselves or others, and indeed a number of studies have shown that the consumption of moderate amounts of alcohol can reduce the risk of heart disease and stroke. But alcohol consumption also has a considerable down side. The acute stage of alcohol intoxication releases normal inhibitions and tends to promote reckless and often violent behaviour. Fights with broken bottles and beer glasses as weapons can interrupt the friendly atmosphere of the

English pub. In addition, the adverse effects of the drug on the regions of the brain that are involved in behaviours that require precise control, as in driving a motor vehicle, make it dangerous to drink and drive. A very high proportion (more than 50 per cent) of fatal traffic accidents are associated with alcohol. A high proportion of violent crimes, in particular domestic violence, are also associated with drinking.

Alcohol's effects at different blood concentrations – according to the British pharmacologist Sir John Gaddum

0.1% – Dizzy and Delightful
0.2% – Drunk and Disorderly
0.3% – Dead Drunk
0.4% – Danger of Death

Stone and Darlington (2000)

A certain proportion of alcohol consumers, perhaps as many as 5–10 per cent, become dependent on the drug as alcoholics. Alcohol will come to dominate their lives, often leading to loss of job and family. They may suffer physical damage to liver (cirrhosis) and other organs, and in extreme cases they may suffer drug-induced brain damage and premature dementia. It is estimated that there are 150,000 alcohol-related deaths in the USA each year.

The consumption of alcohol during pregnancy poses special risks. About 1 in 1,000 of the children born in the USA every year suffer from 'foetal alcohol syndrome'. This is a condition in which the development of the brain is permanently impaired, and it leads to permanent retardation of intellect, with IQ scores of 60 or less. Foetal alcohol syndrome is the single most important cause of mental retardation in the USA. For reasons that are not understood, women differ greatly in their susceptibility to alcohol. As little as 2 units a day can in some cases lead to foetal alcohol syndrome in the baby.

Nicotine

Nicotine is the drug present in tobacco products that is responsible for their pleasurable qualities. The drug acts in the brain on receptors for the chemical messenger acetylcholine. The nerve tracts that release acetylcholine in the brain have among their functions the ability to act as an alerting or arousal system for the cerebral hemispheres – the thinking part of the brain. Smokers say that it helps them to think more clearly and that nicotine has a mild anti-anxiety property.

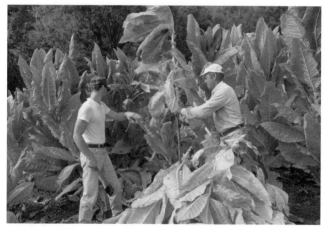

15. Tobacco being harvested in Nashville, Tennessee, USA.

Nicotine is not absorbed well when swallowed, but it can be absorbed by chewing, because of the mildly alkaline conditions in the oral cavity. Nicotine is most efficiently delivered by smoking. The burning tobacco converts the nicotine into a vapour that is inhaled and rapidly absorbed into the blood from the large surface area of the lungs. Smoking delivers nicotine to the brain within seconds of lighting the cigarette. Experienced smokers learn to vary the frequency of puffs and the depth of inhalation to deliver exactly the amount of drug that they want. Unfortunately, smoking also confers special dangers because of the many toxic chemicals present in tobacco smoke. Apart from chemicals already present in the tobacco, new highly toxic cancer-producing chemicals (carcinogens) are created in the process of burning. In addition, cigarette smoke contains an appreciable amount of the gas carbon monoxide (a product of incomplete combustion), which poisons the blood pigment haemoglobin, making it less able to carry oxygen. The latter effect is thought to be one of the principal reasons why mothers who smoke during pregnancy tend to have low birth weight babies – because the foetus is constantly starved of oxygen.

More serious consequences result from the effects of tobacco smoke on the lungs. In the short term these include an increased risk of bronchitis and other forms of obstructive lung disease, and in the longer term an increased risk of lung cancer. The discovery of the link between cigarette smoking and lung cancer was one of the great achievements of medical research of the twentieth century. The initial reports in 1950 from Britain and the USA were followed by many other studies. The findings are alarming: not only is the risk of dying from lung cancer increased in cigarette-smokers, but so are the risks of dying from twenty-three other causes, including cancers of the mouth, throat, larynx, pancreas, and bladder and such obstructive lung diseases as asthma and emphysema. It is hard to overestimate the importance of tobacco smoking as the principal avoidable cause of death in the modern world. More people die from smoking tobacco than any other single cause. Worldwide some three million deaths a year can be attributed to tobacco, and this is likely to rise to ten million a year by the middle of the twenty-first century. In developed countries tobacco is responsible for nearly a quarter of all male deaths and 17 per cent of female deaths. People in the developing countries started smoking later in the twentieth century, but they are catching up fast in the tobacco mortality statistics. The results of a study in China by Liu and colleagues in 1998 involving an analysis of more than one million deaths makes some frightening predictions. Cigarette smoking in China has increased dramatically in the recent past – almost quadrupling since 1980. About two-thirds of men over the age of 25 smoke and about half of these will die before their time. This implies that eventually 100 million of the 300 million young men now alive and aged 0–29 will be killed by tobacco (half dying in middle age, half in old age).

Cigarette smoking first became common among men in the developed world during the early years of the twentieth century, but it was not until thirty or forty years later that the first evidence of a link between tobacco smoking and lung cancer was obtained. Such long lag periods between cause and effect are hard to comprehend. The relationship between cigarette smoking and lung cancer is very complex. The increased risk of developing lung cancer depends far more strongly on the duration of cigarette smoking than on the number of cigarettes consumed each day. Thus, while smoking three times as many cigarettes a day does increase the lung-cancer risk approximately threefold, smoking for thirty years as opposed to smoking for fifteen years does not simply double the lung cancer risk, it increases the risk by twentyfold; and smoking for forty-five years as opposed to fifteen years increases the lung cancer risk one hundredfold.

There are some mitigating features in this otherwise bleak picture. The results of a survey by Doll and Peto in Oxford, published in 2000, show that smokers who quit before they reach the age of 40 suffer only a modest increase in risk of lung cancer. Even for the 50 or 60 year old, giving up smoking conveys a real improvement in such risk. This suggests that more anti-smoking campaigns should be targeted to the adult population and not just to children.

Given the now well-documented health risks associated with smoking, why do so many people continue to indulge in the habit? The answer is that nicotine is a powerfully addictive drug, and users rapidly become dependent – although until recently the tobacco companies have

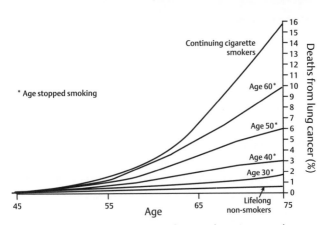

16. The risk of developing lung cancer from smoking cigarettes decreases if smokers quit; the earlier they quit the lower the cancer risk.

strenuously denied this. Some estimates suggest that smoking the first couple of packs of cigarettes carries with it quite a high risk of lifetime dependence. There is a clear psychological withdrawal syndrome experienced by smokers who try to quit – it includes agitation, nervousness, bad temper, and a craving for nicotine. The most successful treatment for smokers trying to quit is to satisfy their craving by administering nicotine by means of chewing gum, skin patches, or a nasal spray. Even with such aids about 80 per cent of those trying to stop smoking will fall back into the habit within six months; without nicotine treatment the figure is more than 90 per cent. Some believe that the reason that smokers need to consume an average of 15–20 cigarettes a day is that they need to keep smoking to stave off the signs of tolerance and withdrawal.

Caffeine

Caffeine, the mild stimulant present in tea and coffee and in cola and other soft drinks, is one of the most widely and frequently consumed drugs in the world. Coffee is second only to oil as an internationally traded commodity and more than ten million people are employed in

Nicotine tolerance and dependence

'The daily smoking cycle can be conceived as follows. The first cigarette of the day produces substantial pharmacological effects, primarily arousal, but at the same time tolerance begins to develop. A second cigarette may be smoked later, at a time when the smoker has learned there is some regression of tolerance. With subsequent cigarettes, there is accumulation of nicotine in the body, resulting in a greater level of tolerance and withdrawal symptoms become more pronounced between successive cigarettes. Transiently high brain levels of nicotine after smoking may partially overcome tolerance. But the primary (euphoric) effects of individual cigarettes tend to lessen throughout the day. Overnight abstinence allows considerable resensitization to the actions of nicotine.'

Benowitz (1990)

its production and marketing. Worldwide the consumption of caffeine is estimated to be approximately 70 mg per person per day – equivalent to a cup of coffee for every person on earth each day. A cup of tea contains on average about half of this amount of caffeine, and a cola drink around 50 mg. There is also a variety of over-the-counter medicines or 'performance-enhancing' drinks that contain larger quantities of caffeine and are recommended to 'relieve tiredness and help maintain mental alertness'.

There have been many studies in human subjects that confirm that caffeine does increase alertness and decrease fatigue. Performance on simple tasks that require sustained attention is improved, and the effect is most marked in subjects whose performance has been impaired by tiredness. Most people seem to be very good at controlling their

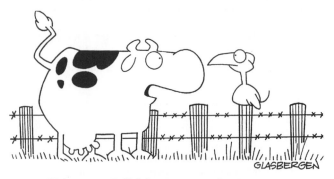

**"It's true, I did jump over the moon.
I had waaaaay too much coffee that day!"**

17.

caffeine consumption to maximize these beneficial effects, taking most caffeine when they require alertness and often avoiding caffeine later in the day to prevent sleep disturbance.

Caffeine acts as an antagonist at receptors in the brain for one of the chemical messengers called adenosine. The adenosine receptors in turn help to regulate the release of a variety of other chemical messengers. One explanation for the stimulant effects of the drug is that by blocking the normal braking actions of adenosine the drug promotes more release of the chemicals acetylcholine and dopamine, both of which have stimulant effects on brain function.

Despite its apparently benign profile, however, there is evidence that chronic caffeine use can lead to a mild form of addiction. Withdrawal of caffeine from regular users leads to increased fatigue, headaches, and impaired performance on simple mental tasks. One school of thought even suggests that one of the reasons why people continue to take coffee, tea, or other caffeine-containing drinks during the day is not so much to improve alertness but to stave off the otherwise unpleasant signs of caffeine withdrawal – in much the same way that

The Vertue of the *COFFEE* Drink.

First publiquely made and sold in England, by *Pasqua Rosee.*

THE Grain or Berry called *Coffee*, groweth upon little Trees, only in the *Deserts of Arabia.*

It is brought from thence, and drunk generally throughout all the Grand Seigniors Dominions.

It is a simple innocent thing, composed into a Drink, by being dryed in an Oven, and ground to Powder, and boiled up with Spring water, and about half a pint of it to be drunk, fasting an hour before, and not Eating an hour after, and to be taken as hot as possibly can be endured; the which will never fetch the skin off the mouth, or raise any Blisters, by reason of that Heat.

The Turks drink at meals and other times, is usually *Water*, and their Dyet consists much of *Fruit*, the Crudities whereof are very much corrected by this Drink.

The quality of this Drink is cold and Dry; and though it be a Dryer, yet it neither heats, nor inflames more then *hot Posset.*

It so closeth the Orifice of the Stomack, and fortifies the heat within, it's very good to help digestion; and therefore of great use to be bout 3 or 4 a Clock afternoon, as well as in the morning.

uch quickens the *Spirits*, and makes the Heart *Lightsome.*

. is good against fore Eys, and the better if you hold your Head o-er it, and take in the Steem that way.

It suppresseth Fumes exceedingly, and therefore good against the *Head-ach*, and will very much stop any *Defluxion of Rheums*, that distil from the *Head* upon the *Stomack*, and so prevent and help *Consumptions*; and the *Cough of the Lungs.*

It is excellent to prevent and cure the *Dropsy, Gout,* and *Scurvy.*

It is known by experience to be better then any other Drying Drink for *People in years*, or *Children* that have any *running humors* upon them, as the *Kings Evil.* &c.

It is very good to prevent *Mis-carryings in Child-bearing Women.*

It is a most excellent Remedy against the *Spleen, Hypocondriack Winds*, or the like.

It will prevent *Drowsiness*, and make one fit for busines, if one have occasion to *Watch*; and therefore you are not to Drink of it *after Supper*, unless you intend to be *watchful*, for it will hinder sleep for 3 or 4 hours.

It is observed that in Turkey, where this is generally drunk, that they are not trobled with the Stone, Gout, Dropsie, or Scurvey, and that their Skins are exceeding cleer and white.

It is neither Laxative nor Restringent.

Made and Sold in St. *Michaels Alley* in *Cornhill*, by *Pasqua Rosee,* at the Signe of his own Head.

18. First known advert for coffee (1660).

cigarette-smokers continue to smoke. Given the widespread and relatively uncontrolled use of caffeine, it is surprising that more research has not been devoted to answering the question of how common caffeine dependence is, or whether it represents a serious public health problem.

Cannabis

Cannabis (known as marijuana in the USA) is the most widely used of all the illegal recreational drugs. Although it has been employed for thousands of years in Asia and the Middle East both as a medicine and as a recreational drug, it is only since the 1960s and 1970s that the recreational use of cannabis has become common in the Western world. As many as a third of the population aged 15–50 in most Western countries will admit to having tried cannabis at least once, and 10–15 per cent of this age group are regular users. The definition of a 'regular user', however, covers a wide range, from those who take the drug every day to those who indulge once a month or less.

Marijuana is the term used to describe the dried leaves and flowering heads of the cannabis plant. The pioneering chemical detective work done by Raphael Mechoulam and his colleagues in the Hebrew University in Jerusalem during the 1970s showed that the principal psychoactive ingredient in the plant is the complex chemical delta-9-tetrahydocannabinol (THC). This accounts for approximately 3–4 per cent of the dry weight of the herbal material, although modern strains of the plant grown indoors under intensive cultivation conditions may contain as much as 15–20 per cent THC. Marijuana is most commonly smoked in cigarettes (joints) or in pipes of various types. Just as cigarette smoking is a very efficient way of delivering nicotine, smoking marijuana delivers THC rapidly to the smoker's brain. By adjusting smoking behaviour, the user can learn to titrate accurately the desired dose of THC. THC is also absorbed when taken by mouth,

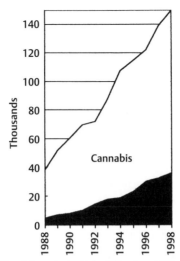

19. Seizures of illegal drugs in the United Kingdom 1988–1998. Seizures of cannabis outweighed those of all other illegal drugs. In 1998 more than 80,000 people were dealt with for cannabis-related offences – which accounted for approximately three-quarters of all drug-related offences.

but this is a less reliable route – the absorption is slow (taking as long as 3–4 hours to reach peak blood levels) and users have no control over whether they will suffer from an overdose or a less than effective dose.

The acute intoxicant effects of cannabis are not unlike those caused by alcohol: users feel a relief of anxiety and often laugh or giggle uncontrollably. Cannabis has its own peculiar effects in distorting the sense of time (so that one minute seems much longer). At high doses it can cause hallucinations and strange fantasies and users can no longer hold a coherent conversation. There is commonly a sudden stimulation of appetite, particularly for sweet foods. These effects may be followed by tiredness and sleep.

A major advance in our understanding of how cannabis works has been the discovery that there is a specific receptor protein in the brain that recognizes THC. But why should nerve cells in our brain possess a receptor that recognizes THC – a chemical found only in the cannabis plant? The answer is that the receptors are there because the brain contains and releases its own THC-like chemical messengers, which normally activate these receptors. The naturally occurring cannabis-like chemicals are fatlike molecules; the principal substance is called 'anandamide', from the Sanskrit word for bliss. These discoveries have had a major impact on the way in which researchers view THC and other cannabinoid drugs. Research in this field started in an attempt to discover how a plant-derived psychoactive drug worked in the brain – but this research has revealed a hitherto unrecognized naturally occurring chemical communication system in the brain. What the normal physiological function of this cannabinoid system is remains unclear, but there are strong clues that among other things it plays an important role in modulating sensitivity to pain.

British Columbia Cannabis Crop

In the endless mountains of British Columbia, on the Gulf Islands scattered along Canada's Pacific Coast, and in countless basements and greenhouses across the province, British Columbia's marijuana trade is booming. No one can say with certainty, but US and Canadian officials and industry insiders put the industry's annual take at $1 billion to $3 billion annually. Much of the crop is destined for markets in the United States. Police estimate that there are some 9,000 growing operations in Vancouver alone, with another thousand in Nanaimo, a medium-sized city a ferry ride away on Vancouver Island. Statements ranking the province's pot business as its second or

The effects on cannabis on pain mechanisms probably underlie the potential medical uses of the drug. Many thousands of patients in the USA and Europe are illicit users of marijuana. They are convinced that the drug treats their symptoms more effectively than any conventional medicine, and they are willing to break the law and to risk arrest and the possibility of stern punishments. The diseases for which patients most commonly report beneficial effects of cannabis are AIDS, multiple sclerosis (MS), spasticity, and various conditions of chronic pain. Patients with AIDS who use marijuana claim in particular that it stimulates appetite and helps to reduce or counteract the loss of body weight. MS patients who use marijuana report that it helps to treat the painful muscle spasms that they frequently suffer. Some forms of chronic pain that do not respond to morphine or other painkillers are also reported to be treatable with marijuana.

Unfortunately there is a woeful lack of scientific evidence to support most of the medical claims for marijuana, although clinical trials in pain and in MS are planned in the UK and may provide the evidence that will lead governments to permit the legal use of cannabis for medical purposes. Moves to legalize such use are already under way in several of the Western States of the USA and in Canada.

Official attitudes to cannabis have not changed since the 1930s, when newspapers in several major American cities ran scare stories about the new 'killer drug'. Alarm about the dangers of marijuana led the US Congress, almost by default, to pass the Marijuana Tax Act in 1937, which effectively banned the further medical use of marijuana and classed it as a dangerous narcotic. This was later reaffirmed by the classification of marijuana in international treaties as a Schedule 1 drug – that is, a dangerous narcotic with no medical uses. This is an even more severe classification than that given to cocaine, heroin, or amphetamines, which do have some legitimate medical uses.

Although there is a large literature on the question of how dangerous a drug cannabis is, it is often confused and lacking in the objectivity we normally expect in science. Nevertheless it is possible to summarize some definite conclusions.

1. It is clear that in the state of acute cannabis intoxication users are not capable of any work that has intellectual demands, and they should not be driving, flying an aeroplane, or operating complex machinery. Unlike alcohol, however, there are virtually no examples of people dying from an overdose of cannabis, nor is there any evidence that the drug provokes aggressive or criminal behaviour.
2. Various alarming scare stories were put forward in the 1970s. It was suggested that marijuana interfered with the secretion of sex hormones in both men and women and might lead to infertility; that the drug impaired the immune system, making people less resistant to infections; and that it might damage the developing foetus. None of these claims has been substantiated by subsequent detailed studies.
3. Long-term regular users of marijuana do show subtle deficits in

higher brain function. In scientific terms we would refer to these as disorders in 'executive brain function' – meaning a reduced ability to remember recent events and to collate and use this information in planning future actions. Such functions are thought to involve regions of the frontal lobe of the brain, an area that is particularly rich in cannabinoid receptors. There have been concerns that these cognitive deficits might persist after marijuana use was stopped – that is, that the drug might cause permanent damage to the brain. But such fears do not appear to be well founded; nearly all of the studies of this topic have found that the cognitive deficits are completely or largely reversible.

4. Why then is marijuana illegal? No drug is completely safe. Marijuana does not kill people, but it is a powerful psychoactive drug and there is increasing evidence that a substantial number of regular users do become dependent on it. A number of studies have found that as many as a third of regular marijuana-users may be classed as 'dependent'. The drug can come to play a dominant role in the lives of large numbers of people – and this is likely to impair their ability to function fully in their work or social life.

5. Perhaps the most serious long-term health hazard in smoking marijuana concerns the risks inherent in the smoke itself. Comparisons of the smoke from marijuana and from tobacco cigarettes have shown that they contain a very similar mixture of toxic chemicals. Marijuana-smokers also inhale more deeply than cigarette-smokers and tend to hold their breath in the mistaken belief that this enhances the absorption of THC in the lungs. As a consequence, marijuana-smokers deposit 4–5 times more tar in their lungs (per joint) than cigarette-smokers. Like tobacco-smokers, marijuana-smokers are liable to develop an irritating cough and signs of bronchitis. There is as yet no evidence that marijuana smoking is associated with an increased risk of lung cancer, but microscopic examination of the cells lining the airways in people who are regular marijuana-smokers has revealed a number of abnormalities suggestive of possible pre-cancerous

changes. The problem in defining the cancer risk is that it may take a very long time for respiratory cancers to reveal themselves. Although a link has not yet been established between marijuana smoking and lung cancer, the habit has been widespread for only a relatively short time in the Western world. As was the case with cigarette smoking, it could take several more decades before any evidence for a link between lung cancer and cannabis smoking became apparent. Meanwhile, we must hope that young people are not storing up a time bomb that may shorten their lives, as tobacco smoking has done for previous generations.

At the beginning of the new millennium we have reached an interesting stage in the cannabis debate in the Western world. We must soon decide whether to reintroduce it into our medicine cabinets, and whether to accept, albeit grudgingly, that the recreational use of cannabis has become part of our culture. Our current official attitude to the drug as a dangerous narcotic comparable to cocaine and heroin is simply not compatible with what we know about the relatively modest hazards of marijuana use.

Morocco: Want Some Weed?

'Every six months, near the start of a new European Union presidency, the Europeans try to discuss their "masterplan for drugs" with Morocco, the world's largest hashish exporter and the supplier of more than 70% of the EU's own intake. To no avail. Morocco's cannabis crop is estimated to earn it over $2 billion a year, the great bulk of the money going to the traffickers – and the officials they bribe. Moreover, it provides an income for Morocco's poorest and unruly regions, the Rif mountains, and sedates its sometimes rebellious 5m Berber

Amphetamines, LSD, and Ecstasy

Amphetamine is one of the first man-made recreational drugs. It was first synthesized in 1887, but was tested in humans only in the 1920s. It was marketed initially as a nasal decongestant (Benzedrine), and also found medical use in the treatment of asthma and as an appetite-suppressant to treat obesity. It is a powerful stimulant though, and the side effect of sleepless nights limited its medical usefulness. This property was precisely the reason that the military started the first non-medical use of the drug during the Second World War, to keep pilots and other military personnel awake and alert during long missions. As a conscript in the British Royal Navy in the 1950s, I found that d-amphetamine (Dexedrine) tablets were still freely available for those on night watch. The dumping of large amounts of surplus amphetamine and the even more potent derivative methamphetamine (Speed) by the American forces in Japan at the end of the war led to the first epidemic of widespread abuse, with up to a million users in Japan in the early 1950s. Some of the consequences soon became apparent, as many heavy users developed a form of madness ('amphetamine psychosis') that closely resembled an acute attack of schizophrenia. Fortunately the drug-induced madness usually proved reversible when drug use was stopped.

Scientifically this turned out to be a very important observation, as the way in which amphetamine acts in the brain is selectively to target those nerve cells that use the messenger molecule dopamine, and to promote an abnormally high rate of release of dopamine in the brain. As we have seen, patients with Parkinson's disease who receive an overdose of L-DOPA can also experience psychotic side effects, and these too are due to an excess of dopamine. The occurrence of amphetamine psychosis in amphetamine addicts helped to point to dopamine as a key to understanding schizophrenic illness, and to the discovery that all effective anti-schizophrenic drugs act as dopamine blockers (see Chapter 3).

Amphetamine abuse spread in Britain and the USA during the 1960s, often associated with cult movements, the 'Mods' in Britain – who used a mixture of amphetamine and barbiturate known as Drinamyl (Purple Hearts) – and motorcycle gangs in the USA – who used methamphetamine (Speed or Crank). The recreational use of amphetamine and methamphetamine is very common, with as many as thirty million regular users worldwide (compared with thirteen million for cocaine and eight million for heroin). A variant has been the use of a methamphetamine-free base ('ice'), a form of the drug that can be smoked. As with many other psychoactive drugs, smoking provides almost instant delivery to the brain and users find this especially pleasurable.

Paradoxically, amphetamine and the amphetamine-like drug methylphenidate (Ritalin) have been found to be useful in treating children with 'attention deficit hyperactivity disorder' (ADHD). These children are hyperactive and cannot attend to anything for more than a short period of time. Consequently they have difficulty in school and usually have poor academic performance. Amphetamine and methylphenidate improve the children's ability to focus their attention and to learn. There is no doubt that these drugs have beneficial effects in some children, although there is a lively debate about whether they are being overprescribed. As many as one American child in ten is said to suffer from some degree of ADHD. There is also the difficult question of whether and when the use of these stimulant drugs can be stopped as children reach adulthood.

Amphetamine is a relatively easy chemical to make – anyone with a basic knowledge of chemistry and the right starting materials can make it in his or her garage or kitchen. It is also fairly easy to make a large number of chemical variants of amphetamine, and several hundred such chemicals have been made and tested in human subjects – so-called designer drugs. One variant is a derivative of methamphetamine, methylene-dioxy-methamphetamine, commonly known as 'Ecstasy'. This is quite an old drug, first launched as a treatment for Parkinson's disease in the 1940s, without any great success. Its popularity as a recreational drug coincided with the rise of the rave dance era of the 1990s. Ecstasy combines the stimulant and alerting effects of amphetamine with euphoriant and mild hallucinogenic properties, probably due to its interaction with serotonin receptors in the brain as well as the dopamine system. Ecstasy was freely available until the mid-1980s, when it was made illegal on both sides of the Atlantic and classified as a Schedule 1 narcotic – that is, a dangerous drug with no medical uses. The properties of the drug are well suited for the rave dance scene – allowing users to stay awake and active all night and inducing a pleasurable feeling of well-being. Following the ban on Ecstasy, a number of the designer amphetamines, which lay for a while outside the legislation, became popular. But Ecstasy has proved more popular than any of these, especially in Western Europe. During the summer of 2000 Ecstasy also became a cult drug for the rave dance scene among young people in the USA. Supplies are readily available from illicit laboratories in Holland and other European countries. Some East European countries have started a new export industry based on supplying Ecstasy to the US market. Several hundred thousand young people use the drug every week. It is not without danger: every year the newspapers carry tragic stories of young people who die as a result of taking the drug. It tends to cause an increase in body temperature and this together with a lack of water or suitable soft drinks can lead to dehydration and death. The number of fatalities is, however, very small by comparison with the widespread consumption of the drug. One has to conclude that it does not warrant the Schedule 1 (dangerous narcotic) classification currently given to it, and this too was the conclusion reached by the UK Police Foundation in its report on drug laws in the United Kingdom published in 2000.

Ecstasy bears a clear chemical resemblance to amphetamine, but it also resembles the hallucinogenic compound mescaline, which is the active ingredient of the mescal cactus, used by Mexican Indians for many centuries in religious rites. Mescaline was discovered by the West as one of the first hallucinogens, and the experience was wonderfully well described by Aldous Huxley (see Box).

Nowadays mescaline has fallen out of favour, but the more potent hallucinogen d-LSD remains very popular. Like Ecstasy, LSD is closely associated with rave dance culture. The drug interacts potently with particular serotonin receptors in the brain to cause intense auditory and visual distortions and hallucinations. It is so powerful that the human dose is about a quarter of one milligram (one-thousandth of a gram). The drug is usually dispensed as a drop of drug solution dried onto a small piece of blotting paper, which is swallowed. There is little evidence that LSD users become dependent on continuing supplies of the drug, but there can be adverse effects. Not all LSD experiences are pleasurable – the 'bad trip' can be an intensely unpleasant and frightening affair. Some users become deluded and may cause their own unintentional injury or death – for example, thinking that they can fly and jumping out of a window.

Aldous Huxley's mescaline experience

'I took my pill at eleven. An hour and a half later I was sitting in my study, looking at a small glass vase. The case contained only three flowers – a full-blown Belle of Portugal rose, shell pink with a hint at every petal's base of a hotter flamier hue; a large magenta and cream-coloured carnation; and, pale purple at the end of its broken stalk, the bold heraldic blossom of an iris. At breakfast that morning I had been struck by the lively dissonance of its colours. But that was no longer the point. I was not looking now at an unusual flower arrangement. I was seeing what Adam had seen on the morning of his creation – the miracle, moment by moment, of naked existence . . . a bunch of flowers shining with their own inner light and all but quivering under the pressure of the significance with which they were charged . . . I continued to look at the flowers, and in their living light I seemed to detect the qualitative equivalent of breathing – but of a breathing without returns to a starting point, with no recurrent ebbs but only a repeated flow from beauty to heightened beauty, from deeper to ever deeper meaning. Words like Grace and Transfiguration came to my mind . . .'

Huxley (1954)

Heroin and cocaine: Dangerous narcotics

In the debate about 'hard' and 'soft' recreational drugs, there is little doubt that heroin and cocaine are regarded as hard drugs. But attitudes in the West have changed over the centuries. As we have seen, opium was widely available and used in the nineteenth century both for medical and for recreational purposes. It was not until late in that century that restriction was first placed on its use, as the problem of addiction was recognized. Cocaine also enjoyed a brief vogue in the 1890s after it was first isolated as a pure compound from coca leaves. Cocaine was incorporated into a number of freely available tonic 'coca-wines' and as an ingredient in the original Coca Cola®, until its dangers were recognized.

Heroin

The powerful natural drug morphine from the opium poppy was a mainstay of medicine for many centuries. Heroin is a synthetic chemical derivative of morphine – it is more potent than the parent drug and it enters the brain from the blood stream more readily. This, together with the preferred route of injecting it into a vein, makes heroin the drug of choice for recreational users. Heroin users describe the 'rush' of intense euphoria and the 'high' that follows intravenous heroin as intensely pleasurable. The intensity of the intravenous heroin high makes heroin use very likely to lead to dependence and physical addiction. Withdrawal from heroin is an unpleasant and potentially life-threatening experience, with liability to diarrhoea, painful stomach cramps, headache, nausea and vomiting, and possibly convulsions. These physical signs are accompanied by an intense craving for the drug. Heroin addiction is an appalling condition: in addition to the hazards inherent in the drug itself, users are likely to die from overdose because the street drug is of variable potency and quality and at high doses the drug depresses respiration; they also run the risk of infection with hepatitis or the AIDS virus HIV because they tend to share the needles used by other addicts to inject the drug. They will develop tolerance and require ever-increasing amounts of the drug to satisfy their craving.

Like morphine, heroin acts on specific 'opiate' receptors in the brain. As in the case of cannabis, these receptors are not there to recognize the plant product. Instead they recognize a family of naturally occurring messenger molecules in the brain, the 'endorphins' (see Chapter 3). There are several different endorphins and at least three distinct types of opiate receptors, but one in particular – the 'mu-opioid receptor' (MOR) seems to be responsible both for the pain-relieving and the pleasurable effects of morphine and heroin. Mice that are genetically engineered so that they do not express MOR in their brain no longer seek out the drug, and it has no pain-relieving actions in such animals.

The use of heroin is unfortunately on the increase, particularly in deprived inner-city areas both in Europe and in the USA. The drug is supplied by well-organized international criminal cartels, using opium from poppies grown as a profitable cash crop in Asia and South America. A modern version of heroin use involves smoking pure heroin as an alternative to injection, a method known as 'chasing the dragon'. Again smoking has proved to be a rapid and effective means of getting the drug quickly to the receptors in the brain – and at least this removes the risk associated with dirty needles.

Treatments for heroin addiction usually involve giving the addict the substitute opiate drug, methadone. This is taken by mouth, is absorbed slowly, and has a long-lasting effect. Without giving the 'high' of heroin it helps to stave off the craving for the drug. Although methadone clinics have had some success, it is difficult to persuade addicts to stop taking heroin. Our society also continues to emphasize the punishment of drug addicts as criminals, rather than as unfortunate individuals in need of medical treatment. To prevent recurrence, the opiate receptor antagonist naltrexone has proved of some use; it prevents the pleasurable effects of the drug. Otherwise programmes of needle exchange, aimed at harm reduction, often seem the best that can be done.

Cocaine

Like morphine, cocaine is a plant product, produced in the leaves of the coca plant – grown particularly in the South American Andes. The huge increase in demand for cocaine as a recreational drug has led to the development of a highly profitable illegal export business for several

South American and Latin American countries. In the case of Colombia, this business has virtually destroyed the fabric of society and the maintenance of law and order.

Chewing coca leaves has been part of everyday life in many South American cultures for centuries; it induces a feeling of well-being, reduces hunger, and increases endurance in an often harsh environment. The peasant chewing coca leaves will obtain only a modest dose of the drug and can adapt to it. The cocaine-user in the Western world, however, is exposed to a pure and far more potent form of the drug. Cocaine is usually taken by insufflating the white powdered cocaine sulphate into the nose, which leads to rapid absorption of the drug into the bloodstream. A modern variant uses a form of cocaine ('crack cocaine'), which is smoked – giving an even more rapid and intensely pleasurable 'high'. Those who have experienced the cocaine high describe it as the most powerful of all drug-induced pleasures. Animals seem to agree (they will rapidly learn to self-administer the drug) and, if given unlimited access, will continue to self-administer to the detriment of all other behaviours – including feeding, drinking, and sex. Cocaine is the ultimate drug of addiction: it is estimated that 10–15 per cent of people who experiment with a snort of cocaine or a smoke of crack cocaine are destined to become regular users, but it is impossible to predict who will succumb in this way. Better to avoid the experiment, as cocaine addiction would seem to be a miserable form of existence. The cocaine high is often followed by a deep depression of mood and the ever-constant need to find the next dose of drug to relieve this black mood. The addict may lack all motivation except to seek further supplies of the drug, and will often steal or murder to obtain these. Cocaine use is fashionable among some professionals – notably journalists and city dealers – but they play a dangerous game.

In the brain cocaine acts to promote both the serotonin and dopamine systems. It does so by acting as an inhibitor of the transporters that are responsible for the uptake of these chemical messengers. This combined pharmacology gives the combined stimulant and arousing effect of amphetamine with the mood-elevating action of Prozac.

Drugs and the law

The regulation of the availability of recreational drugs through legislation has proved to be a very confusing area. While most people would agree that some restrictions need to be placed on the availability of potentially dangerous drugs, particularly to young people, it is less easy to understand why some drugs should be restricted (for example, alcohol) and others banned altogether. Some have described drug taking as a 'victimless crime': who is being damaged other than the users themselves?

Most Western countries have agreed to an international criminal code, which covers many illicit recreational drugs, by means of a series of United Nations conventions framed in the 1960s and 1970s. Most countries operate their own classification system for illicit drugs within this UN framework. In Britain the Misuse of Drugs Act (1971) places drugs in three categories, A, B, and C, with decreasing scales of punishment for criminal offences. The schedules are as follows.

A.   Cocaine, Ecstasy, LSD, morphine, heroin, opium
B.   Amphetamines, barbiturates, cannabis, methamphetamine, codeine
C.   Anabolic steroids, benzodiazepines, pemoline, phentermine, mazindol, diethylpropion

The problem is that, despite the expenditure of large efforts on both sides of the Atlantic in the so-called War on Drugs, the war has not been won. Indeed, the abuse of drugs is continuing to increase and the criminal underworld that supplies this apparently insatiable demand is flourishing. There are no easy solutions in sight. One problem is that the classification of recreational drugs is inappropriate. It suggests, for example, that Ecstasy and cannabis are dangerous narcotic drugs, whereas the weight of scientific evidence now available says that they are not. There are more than half a million cannabis-related arrests in the USA every year, and some 70,000 in Britain – representing in each case around three-quarters of all drug-related offences. Surely police time and resources would be better devoted to really dangerous drugs such as cocaine and heroin? When young people can see that the law is unfair, they come to disrespect it. The Dutch experiment of making small quantities of cannabis freely available in a system of 'coffee shops' has not led to the breakdown of Dutch society – nor do rates of cannabis consumption in Holland differ from those elsewhere in the Western world. The Dutch claim, however, that they have successfully separated the source of cannabis from that of other more dangerous drugs and their problem with heroin and other 'hard drugs' is lessening. In the UK an independent report sponsored by the Police Foundation and published in 2000 agreed with some of these arguments and recommended that cannabis be moved from Category B to Category C, and Ecstasy and LSD from Category A to Category B. The UK government promptly dismissed these suggestions. But sooner or later politicians will have to learn to take the scientific and medical evidence more seriously. Too much of the drug debate has been ill informed and demonized. As a *Lancet* editorial of 11 November 1995 said:

> Cannabis has become a political football, and one that governments continually duck. Like footballs, however, it bounces back. Sooner or later politicians will have to stop running scared and address the evidence: cannabis per se is not a hazard to society but driving it further underground may well be.

Governments can only ignore the views of their electors for so long. A majority of people in most Western countries favour a relaxation of the laws restricting the use of such 'soft drugs' as cannabis and Ecstasy. Furthermore, there is no scientific justification for classifying such drugs as dangerous narcotics. Sooner or later the majority view will prevail and changes in the drug laws will occur, making them more rational and in tune with modern culture. By 2020 we may be as puzzled that these changes took so long to happen as we were in past decades that the reform of the laws governing homosexual behaviour came only after they were long overdue.

Chapter 5
Making new medicines

The discovery, development, and marketing of new prescription
medicines has become a major worldwide industry. Pharmaceutical
companies, focused mainly in the USA, Western Europe, and Japan, have
become an important component of the economies of many developed
nations. Some of the individual companies are among the largest and
wealthiest in any industry, employing tens of thousands of staff and
enjoying annual revenues amounting to many billions of dollars. The
successful discovery and marketing of a new medicine can also be a very
profitable business, with annual sales of 'blockbuster' drugs often in
excess of $1 billion and carrying a high profit margin. Such returns are
always transitory though; there will always be a competitor coming
along with a similar medicine willing to undercut in price. The
pharmaceutical industry relies heavily on patents to protect its
products, so that a competitor cannot immediately sell the same
medicine, but a competitor can market a similar product that lies
outside the scope of the original patent. Patents also have finite lives
and the twenty years of protection provided by a patent are often
substantially eroded during the long process of research and
development (R&D) needed before a product can come to market. After
the patent expires, any company can copy the drug and market it as a
so-called generic product, and this has created a secondary industry of
companies that specialize in the production and marketing of generic
medicines. As they do not have to incur the expensive costs of R&D, the

generic drug companies can market the product much more cheaply than the original discoverer. Because new products have only a finite commercial life, the major companies must always be looking for the next generation of medicines, preferably the new blockbusters. How this is done has become an extraordinarily complex and high-tech process.

Drug discovery

All drugs act on specific receptors (see Chapter 2) and most innovative companies seek to discover new receptor targets that offer a novel approach to the treatment of a particular disease. The range of new targets available is being extended greatly as our knowledge of the human genome becomes increasingly complete. Humans have around 30,000–40,000 genes, each of which encodes the information for making a protein. Clearly not all of these will be suitable drug targets, but many new targets will emerge. All the medicines that are available in 2001 target less than 2,000 different receptors, so this number will undoubtedly increase. The problem for companies is how to decide which of the many possible novel receptors offer the greatest chance of providing effective new treatments, and which ones to invest in. The choice of new drug discovery targets is thus now associated with an embarrassment of riches. New targets will, nevertheless, be found that offer novel approaches to treating diseases, based on new knowledge of the disease process.

Once a target has been chosen, the human target protein can be made or expressed in immortalized cell cultures so that it is available for the testing of large numbers of new drug candidates. The synthesis of new drug chemicals as candidates for such screening used to be a laborious and slow process. Each new chemical was made individually by expert chemists, who on average could produce one or two new compounds each week. Since the 1990s, however, this process has been radically changed by the introduction of robot chemistry, which allows the assembly of the various chemical constituents that make up new drug molecules in many different permutations. Using such 'combinatorial chemistry' techniques, a single chemist can now produce thousands of new compounds each week. Specialized companies have emerged that synthesize chemical libraries containing hundreds of thousands or even millions of new chemicals and sell them to pharmaceutical companies for their own particular screening projects. The screening of large numbers of new chemicals has become possible because of the parallel development of new 'high throughput' screening technology. By using robot laboratories capable of handling very large numbers of tests and using computers to store the mass of data that result, it is now possible for a company to screen as many as a million new chemicals in less than one month against a given target. Often these chemical libraries are made up of a random selection of many different types of molecules, but sometimes more selective libraries are prepared, based on molecules that somewhat resemble the natural receptor agonist or enzyme substrate or that mimic already available drugs. This process of mass screening should generate a number of 'lead' chemicals with some activity at the target receptor. By examining the chemical features that the lead structures have in common, chemists can then further refine these leads to create improved drug candidates with even stronger actions on the target receptor.

The large-scale screening involves simple tests on the human receptor target in a test tube or cell culture model. The next stage will involve testing the best drug candidates in more complex biological systems, often using the isolated organs or tissues of experimental animals – whose receptor proteins are usually very similar to their human counterparts. The short-listed candidates may then be tested by giving them to living animals. In some cases this is the only way of testing the effectiveness of new drug candidates – for example in assessing the effects of drugs on animal behaviour in tests that predict new antidepressant or anti-schizophrenic medicines.

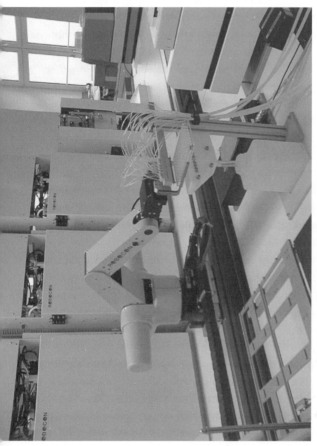

20. Laboratory robot, seen here holding a 96-well plastic plate in its me mass screening of large numbers of test compounds in laboratory tests new drug molecules. Such machines can work night and day 7 days a thousands of new chemicals each day.

Drug development

The initial screening may involve hundreds of thousands of chemicals, but this will have been reduced to a short list of 10–100 candidates for assessment in the whole-animal tests. From these, a handful of possible development candidates will emerge. Each of these needs to be assessed to see whether it is likely to provide a useful and safe medicine. Further animal experiments will be needed to establish how well the compounds are absorbed when given by mouth and how long their actions last. A compound that is not well absorbed when given by mouth will be troublesome unless another route of administration can be devised. One that is well absorbed but rapidly degraded or eliminated will also not be attractive, as in human use this would mean that the patient would have to take several doses each day.

To obtain approval for the introduction of a new medicine, the company needs to satisfy the various government regulatory agencies both that the compound is effective in treating the condition for which it is intended and that it is unlikely to be dangerous to the patient. The safety of new drugs can never be fully predicted by tests in animals, but these can at least eliminate many potentially toxic substances. All governments require extensive animal safety testing. This involves, for example, testing the potential new medicine by administering it to animals at various doses, including at least one high dose greatly in excess of any planned human use. The drug is administered every day for periods of up to twelve months. During this period the animals will be weighed regularly and blood samples taken to see whether any biochemical or blood abnormalities are triggered. At the end of the test period the animals are killed and their various internal organs visually examined and weighed and then examined in detail under the microscope to detect any possible adverse changes. These safety tests will be repeated in two different mammalian species to maximize the chance of detecting any toxicity. Special animal tests in pregnant animals will be needed if the drug is to be used in women of child-bearing age – to detect any possible adverse effects that the compound might have on the developing foetus (the thalidomide tragedy was the spur to improve such tests). Other safety tests will be undertaken using both simple models and whole animals to see whether the new compound is likely to cause or to stimulate the growth of cancers. Any drug that is to be used over a substantial period of time in humans will have to be tested for cancer liability in animal tests lasting two years in two different animal species.

Clinical trials

Provided the development compound passes these safety tests, it can then be administered to human subjects for the first time. The initial Phase 1 clinical trials involve a small number of healthy volunteers. They receive the drug under carefully monitored conditions to make sure that it does not cause any unpredicted unpleasant or dangerous side effects. Monitoring drug levels in blood samples from such volunteers will also provide valuable information on how well the drug is absorbed in humans, how long it persists in the body, and what the main breakdown products are. This information will help the selection of the most suitable dose regime for the next stage (Phase 2) of clinical tests, which involve patients. These trials are usually done with small numbers of patients, and the aim is to test whether the drug actually works – that is, does it improve the patients' symptoms? In the case of drugs that target a novel human receptor for the first time, this 'proof of concept' is particularly vital; it may not always work out the way the scientists predicted. For example, a few years ago my colleagues at Merck & Co. Inc. discovered a drug that blocked the receptors for the brain peptide cholecystokinin (CCK). CCK itself had previously been found to cause brief but unpleasant panic attacks when injected intravenously in human volunteers. The new drug was able completely to prevent this chemically induced panic state. It seemed logical, therefore, to undertake clinical trials to see whether the CCK-blocker might be useful in treating the symptoms of panic in patients who are unfortunate enough to suffer from recurrent panic attacks. After several weeks of drug treatment, however, it was clear that the drug was of no benefit at all to such patients, who continued to suffer regular panic attacks as before. Nice try – but the logic was weak: 'CCK causes panic, therefore panic is caused by CCK' is a non-sequitur.

All clinical trials need to take account of the 'placebo' effect. Sick patients want to believe that the new medicine will help them to get better, and it is well established that many patients show a definite measurable improvement even when given a dummy (placebo) pill that does not contain any active drug. The placebo effect is particularly marked for disorders of the central nervous system; trials of new antidepressants or pain-relieving compounds will always show a placebo effect. The nature of the placebo effect remains a mystery. The strength of the placebo effect is related to the complexity of the treatment procedure. Swallowing several tablets has a more powerful effect than simply taking one, an intravenous injection is even more powerful, and treatment involving a mock surgical procedure is even better. As with many drug treatments, the effectiveness of the placebo tends to wear off with repeated administrations. The placebo effect seems to reflect the remarkable ability of the human mind to control the body, and it may well underlie the effectiveness of various 'alternative-medicine' approaches to treating illness. From the point of view of drug development, however, the placebo effect complicates the clinical assessment of new drugs. In order to see whether any beneficial effects observed in patients are due to the drug itself or simply to a placebo effect, it is necessary to compare the active drug with a placebo. This is usually accomplished in a so-called randomized double-blind placebo controlled trial. In such trials patients are randomly allocated to groups that receive either a placebo or an active drug. Neither the patient nor the doctor nor nurse administering the medicine knows whether the patient is receiving an active drug or a placebo – to avoid any possibility of suggestion. At the end of the trial the code is broken and the results analysed. Only if the drug is statistically significantly more beneficial than the placebo can the trial be called a success. The results of these trials will also help to establish whether the drug caused any adverse side effects over and above any that were observed in the placebo group. For example, it is common for patients to complain of headache or feelings of nausea, but these may not necessarily be drug related. If adverse drug-related effects are observed, these must be noted and explained to all patients receiving the compound in the future.

In the happy event that the results of the Phase 2 trials are positive, the compound can enter much larger Phase 3 clinical trials. These commonly involve thousands of patients, recruited in a number of different medical centres – usually university medical schools and hospitals. Because of their complexity, and the need to treat patients over extended periods of time, these trials can often take years to complete. At every stage detailed records need to be kept of each patient and, wherever possible, objective methods used to measure improvement in clinical state. One may measure reductions in blood pressure or blood cholesterol, for example. In some conditions, however, particularly those involving disorders of the central nervous system, such objective measurements may not be possible – and one has to rely on the patients' own assessments of their mood, or how much pain they are feeling.

Registration and marketing

If all goes well with these Phase 3 trials, the company will be ready to assemble a massive package of data. This will include a detailed description of all the results obtained on the compound in the clinic, in animal safety and in the laboratory, together with information on how the compound can be manufactured and what quality-control measures exist. Such a package of data will occupy many volumes, enough to fill several very large bookcases. It will be submitted to a government regulatory agency for detailed scrutiny, and after expert assessment the agency will inevitably come back to the company with a list of questions that need to be answered, often involving the need for the company to undertake further tests for efficacy or safety. After this process has been completed the agency may hold a public meeting at which a panel of experts can interrogate company representatives on the fine points of their submission. The panel then votes to advise the government agency whether to approve or decline the submission. The process of review by the regulatory agency can take years to complete, although for some diseases (for example, AIDS) there are fast-track approval procedures.

Once a new medicine has been given official registration, the company is free to market it, but it can only be recommended and advertised for the particular disorders for which official approval was given. Any additional new medical uses will need further clinical trial data and government approval before the company can promote these. After marketing has started there is a system of 'post-marketing surveillance', which requires doctors to alert the authorities to adverse drug effects. This is designed to detect any rare adverse effects that the compound may cause. Even though the clinical trials involve thousands of patients, they cannot detect rare adverse effects that may occur, for example, in only 1 in 100,000 patients. These can sometimes be serious or even life threatening, and they can lead to the rapid withdrawal of new compounds from the market – a bitter pill to swallow for the company involved. New medicines represent entirely novel chemical molecules to which humans have never been exposed; their safety is never going to be completely predictable.

The complex and exacting process of drug discovery and development takes many years to complete and involves company scientists and outside experts from many different disciplines. The whole process from initial screening to final product often takes ten years or more and the costs involved continue to escalate as regulatory agencies set more and more demanding criteria for drug approval. On average, for every

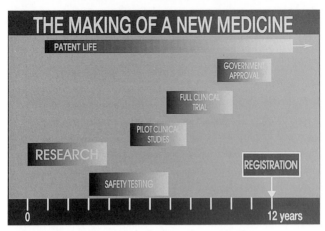

THE MAKING OF A NEW MEDICINE

PATENT LIFE

GOVERNMENT APPROVAL

FULL CLINICAL TRIAL

PILOT CLINICAL STUDIES

RESEARCH

REGISTRATION

SAFETY TESTING

0

12 years

21. The making of a new medicine involves a number of time-consuming stages. Overall the process from laboratory bench to doctor's desk can take more than 10 years.

100 promising drug candidates discovered in the research laboratory only ten will get as far as being assessed in human subjects, and only one of these will become a registered new medicine. Even then, less than half of the new medicines will make a profit for the company. Since each new medicine costs several hundred million dollars to develop, pharmaceutical companies use the high cost of R&D to justify the high prices and profit margins they obtain for new products. This is partly justified, as the remarkable success of the pharmaceutical industry in discovering innovative new treatments for human disease depends on the ability to spend heavily on R&D. Pharmaceutical companies reinvest more than 10 per cent of their income on R&D, a far higher proportion than most other sectors of industry. On the other hand, the companies make very high profit margins, and they spend equally heavily on marketing their products, both to doctors and more recently to the individual patient. Stock markets rate pharmaceutical companies' shares very highly, and expect the income of the major companies to

continue to grow in double-digit figures every year. For an industry that depends heavily on products with a limited patent life, this means that there is an intense pressure to find the next blockbuster drug. Those companies that fail to do so may merge or be absorbed by others who have been more successful. Each year sees the industry increasingly dominated by a smaller number of giant companies formed as the result of such mergers. The high prices that new prescription medicines command, and the profits that companies report, have given the pharmaceutical industry a poor public image in recent years. There is anger too about the fact that poor countries are denied the benefits of Western medicines, because the industry insists on maintaining the patent restrictions on its products throughout the world. Although governments already exert considerable regulation over the industry, for example, in setting new product prices in many countries, it seems likely that there will be pressure for even more such intervention in the future.

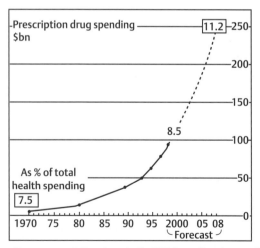

22. Spending on prescription drugs in the USA is predicted to continue to rise rapidly.

Prescription medicines are not the only medicines on the market. It is far easier to gain approval for the introduction of herbal medicines where proof of efficacy is not required. On the other hand, the company marketing a herbal medicine is also not allowed to make specific medical claims for it; the alleged benefits have to be couched in more general terms. Homeopathic medicines represent a special case, as these often involve diluting active ingredients to such an extent that there may be few or no active drug molecules remaining in the marketed preparation, the ultimate placebo medicine. Regulatory agencies have never been sure how to deal with homeopathic medicines. At the end of the day they seem to have concluded that at least they are unlikely to do patients any serious harm and their approval remains relaxed.

Chapter 6

The twentieth century and beyond

In 1900 aspirin had just been launched; by 2000 it had been joined by many thousands of other new medicines. The pace and scale of these advances not only changed the way in which medicine is practised; they have changed all of our lives.

Tuberculosis: the 'white death'

In 1900 half of all deaths in the USA were due to infectious diseases, and of these tuberculosis was the most important, accounting for 11 per cent of all deaths in that year. One hundred years earlier in the overcrowded slums of Victorian cities tuberculosis was even more deadly. Death from tuberculosis was so common it was even romanticized by early Victorian poets, artists, and novelists, who depicted consumptives as young, beautiful, innocent, and frequently female. Although improvements in housing, nutrition, and hygiene helped reduce tuberculosis mortality, it was not until the introduction of the first effective medicines in the latter half of the twentieth century that the disease was finally conquered.

The tuberculosis bacterium – *Mycobacterium tuberculosis* – is an unusual organism. It is very resistant to the normal white cell defences of the immune system. When the tuberculosis bacteria are engulfed by scavenging white cells, they do not always die; indeed they may kill the white cells. The body activates other defences, surrounding clusters of the invading bacteria with a wall of granular tissue to prevent further spread. The bacteria within such granulomas grow very slowly or can remain dormant for years before being reactivated. The lungs are often the primary site of attack, but the bacteria can spread to bone, joints, and spinal cord. The unfortunate patient grows gradually weaker with pustulant infectious foci often erupting to the surface of the body.

The first effective drug treatment was discovered in the 1940s by Selman Waksman at Rutgers University in New Jersey. It had long been known that the tubercle bacillus was rapidly inactivated in the ground. In a sample of soil he discovered a new strain of fungus that made the powerful antibiotic streptomycin, the first found to be effective in treating tuberculosis (a discovery that earned him the Nobel Prize for Physiology and Medicine in 1952). Streptomycin was developed and marketed by Merck & Co in the early 1950s, following their experience in producing penicillin by large-scale fermentation techniques during the Second World War. Streptomycin was rapidly followed by other effective drugs, para-amino-salicylic acid (PASA), a close chemical relative of aspirin (Figure 11), and isoniazid, another synthetic chemical. Use of these drugs, often in a 'triple therapy' combination, radically changed the treatment of the disease, often literally rescuing patients from their deathbeds and effectively removing tuberculosis as a major cause of death in the Western world.

There is little room for complacency, however, as new drug-resistant strains of *Mycobacterium tuberculosis* emerged in the 1980s and 1990s in the Third World, where tuberculosis remains an important killer disease. These drug-resistant strains have also appeared in deprived areas of Western cities and the number of new cases of the disease showed a worrying increase in the West during the 1990s. More research is urgently needed to provide new anti-tuberculosis drugs. Some grounds for hope for the future exist. The entire genome (DNA sequence) of

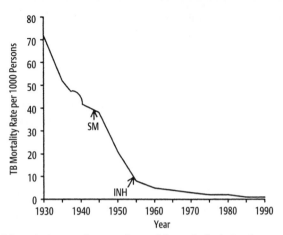

23. Tuberculosis mortality rates dropped dramatically during the twentieth century, speeded by the development of effective drug treatments in the 1950s. SM = streptomycin, INH = isoniazid.

Mycobacterium tuberculosis is now known, and this should provide scientists with new targets to attack.

The discovery of effective treatments for tuberculosis was only one of many twentieth-century triumphs in the ongoing battle against infectious diseases. We take antibiotics for granted nowadays, and we do not expect to die from infectious diseases, which by the end of the twentieth century were responsible for less than 5 per cent of deaths in the USA, compared to more than 50 per cent in 1900. The advent of the first effective treatments for HIV/AIDS within a mere decade after the disease was first recognized is another remarkable achievement, although the drugs remain far too expensive to be used in poor countries where many of the thirty million people infected with HIV live. This highlights an ever-increasing concern that the poor countries of the world are denied access to the fruits of medical research.

Tuberculosis in Victorian England

'There is a dread disease which so prepares its victim, as it were, for death . . . a dread disease, in which the struggle between soul and body is so gradual, quiet and solemn, and the results so sure, that day by day, and grain by grain, the mortal part wastes and withers away, so that the spirit grows light . . . a disease in which death and life are so strangely blended that death takes the glow and hue of life, and life the gaunt and grisly form of death – a disease which medicine never cured, wealth warded off, or poverty could boast exemption from – which sometimes moves in giant strides, or sometimes at a tardy sluggish pace, but, slow or quick, is ever sure and certain.'

Charles Dickens, *Nicholas Nickleby*

Oral contraceptives

Oral contraceptives represent another example of twentieth-century drugs that have changed our lives. They have certainly changed women's lives, making motherhood a matter of choice rather than necessity and thus liberating them from a lifetime of child-bearing. Gregory Pincus, working in Worcester, Massachusetts, discovered the first effective oral contraceptive. Pincus knew that raised levels of the female sex hormone progesterone during pregnancy prevented ovulation (the release of mature egg cells from the ovary). He found that treating rabbits with large doses of progesterone prevented them from becoming pregnant. Clinical trials with a synthetic progesterone-like chemical, norethylnodrel, were undertaken in 1958 in Puerto Rico. None of the 221 fertile women enrolled in the trial became pregnant, and the first oral contraceptive pill was launched in 1960. Since then there have been many refinements. Most oral contraceptives nowadays contain a mixture of a progesterone-like chemical and an oestrogen-like substance (oestrogen is the second female sex hormone). The pill seeks to mimic the hormonal conditions in the woman's body during early pregnancy.

Oral contraceptives are highly effective: when taken regularly, they are almost 100 per cent effective in protecting against pregnancy. Their almost universal use in the Western world has dramatically altered sexual and reproductive behaviour. The sexual revolution of the 1960s would not have been possible without the contraceptive pill. The ability to choose when to have a baby has led increasing numbers of women to defer child-bearing until later in life, when they have established their careers. Child-bearing in women in their late thirties or early forties is no longer uncommon. For politicians, this freedom of choice poses a new and unexpected set of problems for the future. Most West European countries are already in a state of negative population growth. Every ten women in Spain, for example, will during their lifetime bear only eleven children. Western Europe as a whole can expect to see its population fall from the present 350 million to less than 300 million by the year 2050. The impact of these trends is made more severe because Western countries have an increasingly aged population – the ratio of those in work to pensioners could fall from its present figure of 4:1 to less than 2:1 by 2050.

Age-related diseases

The availability of effective treatments for infectious diseases, and the widespread use of increasingly effective treatments for high blood pressure and heart disease, are among the many factors underlying the tendency of people in the Western world to live longer. The over-85 age group is among the fastest growing of any sector of the population in Europe and the USA. The number of centenarians in Britain has risen from around 200 in 1920 to more than 10,000 today, and the numbers are doubling every ten years. By 2050 we could have more than 50,000 centenarians in Britain – one for every 1,000 people! These figures should be a cause for celebration, but they also mean that the health services will have to cope with an ever-increasing number of people with age-related diseases.

Among these are disorders of the body, the joints, muscles, and bladder – but perhaps the most insidious are the age-related degenerative diseases of the brain. The biggest problem of all is Alzheimer's disease. It affects around 10 per cent of all those over the age of 65, and this rises to 25 per cent or more of those over the age of 80. Alzheimer's disease has been known for more than 100 years, since Alois Alzheimer first described the characteristic pathological changes that occur in the brains of Alzheimer's patients. But it is still a poorly understood disease. It is characterized by abnormal protein deposits that accumulate in the brain and lead eventually to a massive loss of brain cells. This in turn causes intellectual impairment, and ultimately physical disability and death. The dementia associated with Alzheimer's disease is particularly distressing for those who care for the patient. The patients lose memory and intellectual function and have little insight into their illness; they are unable to recognize close family or friends; they may develop unpleasant and distressing psychotic and aggressive behaviour, and yet at first show little or no sign of physical illness.

New knowledge about the biochemical basis of the disease has been gained, and this will hopefully lead to treatments that will arrest or slow the downwards progress of the illness, but these advances are still many years ahead. Meanwhile the only effective drugs are those that boost the function of the monoamine acetylcholine in the brain. The acetylcholine-containing nerves, which play an important role in memory and other cognitive brain functions, are among the first to degenerate in the Alzheimer's brain. The cholinergic drugs (for example, Aricept® and Rivastil®) can provide modest improvements in memory and other intellectual functions at least for a while, although they do not affect the underlying progressive degenerative process.

Cancer

There has been an enormous basic medical research effort devoted to understanding the biochemical changes that occur in normal body cells to turn them into cancer cells that grow in an uncontrolled manner and aggressively invade various parts of the body. While major scientific advances have come from this research, what they have told us is that there are many different biochemical mechanisms that can lead to cancer; there is no single underlying cause. This makes cancer particularly hard to treat, as each type of cancer is different. Since 1950 great progress has been made in treating some forms of cancer, while others remain largely untreatable. For example, testicular cancer in men is now largely treatable with anti-cancer drugs – with better than 90 per cent success rates. The same is true for Hodgkin's disease, a cancer of the lymph nodes. For lung cancer and other similar fast-growing cancers, however, there are essentially no effective treatments.

In terms of drug treatment, most of the present-day drugs are ones that attack rapidly growing cells and kill them. They inevitably cause damage to some of the normal cells of the body and lead to severe and unpleasant side effects. The most powerful anti-cancer drugs are based on the platinum-containing drug cisplatin, or on the compound taxol extracted from yew-tree leaves. The use of these powerful drugs is limited partly by their propensity to cause severe nausea and vomiting. These unpleasant side effects can, however, nowadays be treated effectively with a new generation of anti-nausea drugs that act on one of the receptors for the monoamine serotonin in the vomiting centre in the brain. The 5-HT_3 receptor antagonists have radically improved the treatment of cancer patients in recent years.

Looking to the future, the treatment of cancers will undoubtedly be improved, as more and more biological agents become available. The medical use of monoclonal antibodies is still in its infancy, but many such products are under development for the selective targeting of cancer cells. Herceptin is one such compound launched in 1999 for the treatment of breast cancer – it specifically targets and neutralizes a protein herpin that is produced by some forms of breast cancer and is needed for the cancer to grow. Other drugs in development target biochemical targets that are unique to the cancer cell. For example, the enzyme telomerase is not found in normal adult human cells, but it is switched on in cancer cells; it allows them to divide indefinitely, which normal cells cannot. Telomerase inhibitors could offer a selective way of attacking cancerous cells.

Another exciting future prospect is to employ gene therapy. Here the idea is to use DNA itself as a drug, carrying the information needed to make a protein that will help the body fight illness. People who have an inherited defect in a particular protein could be treated with DNA that will allow them to make the correct protein. One approach to gene therapy in cancer has been to attempt to introduce the gene for a drug-metabolizing enzyme selectively into cancer cells; they would then be able to convert a harmless pro-drug into a lethal cell poison, and the pro-drug could be administered safely, as the other cells in the body would be unable to undertake this lethal conversion. So far attempts at gene therapy have proved disappointing – the main problem being how to deliver the DNA efficiently into the cells where it is needed.

Future gazing

In the wake of the unravelling of the human genome, prospects have never looked brighter for the biomedical sciences. It is possible that most of the remaining intractable human illnesses will see major advances leading to treatments in the next few decades. The application of monoclonal antibodies and other therapeutic proteins will increase dramatically, and ways will be found to solve the delivery problems that have so far prevented gene therapy.

One problem that may limit the widespread application of these medical benefits, however, will be their cost. Monoclonal antibodies and other therapeutic proteins are far more costly to manufacture than old-fashioned chemical drug molecules. The companies making them are also hungry for profits. A single dose of monoclonal antibody can cost thousands of dollars. The extreme example of costly biologicals has already been seen with the treatment of a rare inherited disease, Gaucher's disease, which affects the development of the brain. By injecting children suffering from the disease with an enzyme that restores normal brain biochemistry, a dramatic improvement in their quality of life is possible. But the treatment has to be repeated at regular intervals and it costs about $250,000 per patient each year. Fortunately this is a rare disease, and US medical insurance companies have so far been willing to pay. But will countries that are not as rich as the USA be able to afford to keep up? Prescription drug spending in the USA is predicted to double from the a level of around $100 billion per year in 2000 to more than US$200 billion by 2010. But, there are already pressures to restrict prescription drug spending in most European countries, and the Third World hardly has access at all to modern Western medicines except through piracy and by ignoring the patent laws. The biotechnology and pharmaceutical industries may ironically become victims of their own success in the twenty-first century, as an increasing number of health services find that they cannot afford to use all the expensive goods on offer.

References

Chapter 1

Berridge, V., and Edwards, G. (1981), *Opium and the People* (London: St Martin Press, Allen Lane).

Culpepper, N. (1770), *The English Physician Enlarged. With 369 Medicines made of English Herbs* (London).

Encyclopaedia Britannica (2000), 'Medicine – History of: Medicine and Surgery before 1800': www.britannica.com

Hoffmann, A. (1994), 'History of the Discovery of LSD', in A. Pletscher and D. Ladweig (eds.), *50 Years of LSD* (London: Parthenon Publishing Group).

Chapter 3

IMS Health World Review (2000): www.imshealth.com

UK House of Lords (1997), Select Committee on Science and Technology, *Report on 'Resistance to Antibiotics'* (London: HMSO).

Chapter 4

Benowitz, N. L. (1990), *The Biology of Nicotine Dependence* (CIBA Foundation Symposium 152; Chichester: John Wiley & Sons).

Huxley, A. (1954), *The Doors of Perception* (London: Chatto and Windus).

Liu, B. Q., *et al.* (1998), 'Emerging Tobacco Hazards in China. I:

Retrospective Proportional Mortality Study of One Million Deaths',
British Medical Journal, 317: 1411–22.

Peto, R., *et al.* (2000), Smoking, Smoking Cessation, and Lung Cancer in
the UK since 1950: Combination of National Statistics with Two Case
Control Studies', *British Medical Journal*, 321: 323–9.

Smith, P. (2000), *Drug Reform Coordination Network*: psmith@drcnet.org

Stone, T., and Darlington, G. (2000), *Pills, Potions, and Poisons* (Oxford:
Oxford University Press).

UK Police Foundation (2000), *Report of the Independent Inquiry into the
Misuse of Drugs Act 1971* 'Drugs and the Law' (London: The Police
Foundation).

Further reading

Pharmacology and the medical uses of drugs

Cooper, J., Bloom, F. E., and Roth, R.H., *The Biochemical Basis of Neuropharmacology* (7th edn., Oxford: Oxford University Press, 1996). Excellent introductory student text on drugs that act on the nervous system.

Hardman, J. G., and Imbard, L. (eds.) *Goodman & Gilman's the Pharmacological Basis of Therapeutics* (9th edn., New York: McGraw Hill, 1996). The definitive textbook.

Healy, D., *The Antidepressant Era* (Cambridge, Mass.: Harvard University Press, 1997). A fascinating account of the history of antidepressant drugs in the twentieth century, written for the non-specialist reader.

Karlen, A. *Plagues Progress: A Social History of Man and Disease* (London: Victor Gollancz, 1995). A good account of how infectious diseases have influenced history.

Stone, T., and Darlington, G., *Pills, Potions and Poisons: How Drugs Work* (Oxford: Oxford University Press, 2000). An introductory book written for the non-specialist reader.

Non-medical uses of drugs

Iversen, L., *The Science of Marijuana* (New York: Oxford University Press, 2000). A review of how cannabis works and the pros and cons of its medicinal or recreational use, written for the non-specialist.

Jay, M. (2000), *Emperors of Dreams: Drugs in the Nineteenth Century* (Sawtry, Cambs.: Dedalus, 2000). A well-written account of the social history of recreational drug use in the nineteenth century, from laughing gas and ether to heroin and cocaine.

Regan, Ciaran, *Intoxicating Minds* (London: Weidenfeld & Nicolson, 2000). An engaging account of mind-altering drugs in history and an explanation of how they work in the brain.

Robson, P., *Forbidden Drugs* (2nd edn., Oxford: Oxford University Press, 1999). Readable account of recreational drugs and drug abuse.

Drugs

Index

Drugs

Visit the
VERY SHORT
INTRODUCTIONS
Web site

www.oup.co.uk/vsi

➤ **Information** about all published titles

➤ News of **forthcoming books**

➤ **Extracts** from the books, including titles
not yet published

➤ **Reviews** and views

➤ **Links** to other **web sites** and main
OUP web page

➤ Information about **VSIs in translation**

➤ **Contact** the editors

➤ **Order** other **VSIs** on-line